NATURAL ALTERNATIVES To LIPITOR, ZOCOR & other Statin Drugs

JAY S. COHEN, MD

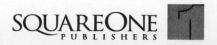

SQUAREONE
PUBLISHERS

The information and advice contained in this book are based upon the research and the personal and professional experiences of the author. They are not intended as a substitute for consulting with a healthcare professional. The publisher and author are not responsible for any adverse effects or consequences resulting from the use of any of the suggestions, preparations, or procedures discussed in this book. All matters pertaining to your physical health should be supervised by a healthcare professional. It is a sign of wisdom, not cowardice, to seek a second or third opinion.

COVER DESIGNER: Jeannie Tudor
IN-HOUSE EDITOR: Elaine Weiser
TYPESETTER: Gary A. Rosenberg

Square One Publishers
115 Herricks Road
Garden City Park, NY 11040
516-535-2010 • 877-900-BOOK
www.squareonepublishers.com

CONTENTS

NATURAL ALTERNATIVES VS. STATIN DRUGS

Cardiovascular disease has been the leading cause of death in the United States and the developed world for many decades. Each year in America, coronary artery disease causes 1.1 million heart attacks and 515,000 deaths. More than 700,000 people suffer strokes; 167,000 die, and many of the survivors remain permanently disabled.[1] Yet despite decades of research, controversy about the causes, treatment, and prevention of cardiovascular disease continues. Many doctors believe that cholesterol is the main culprit, and that an elevated cholesterol level automatically means treatment with one of the statin drugs (Lipitor, Zocor, Crestor, Mevacor, Pravachol, Lescol). So it is no surprise that statins are the most prescribed drugs in America, and that Lipitor is the most prescribed drug of all. Some doctors are so enthusiastic about statins' ability to reduce cholesterol levels, they call statins "miracle drugs," claim that statins cause no side effects, and state that everyone over age forty should be taking a statin.

Fortunately, many patients are not as eager to take statin drugs for the rest of their lives as their doctors are to prescribe them. Survey results have shown that nearly two-thirds of adults avoid taking prescription drugs whenever possible. In addition, many patients have questions that should be answered before drugs are dispensed. This applies especially to the use of statin drugs, but too often these questions go unanswered. This book will answer the following questions (and many more) in helping you decide whether you require cholesterol reduction and, if so, whether you might use a natural alternative instead of a statin medication.

- Do I need to lower my cholesterol level? If so, how much?

- What about the good HDL-cholesterol? Should it be higher?

- What about the other risk factors for heart disease?

- Do I need to take a statin drug?

- Are there effective natural therapies I can use instead?

- How do the natural therapies differ? Can they be used in combination or with a statin drug?

- Are there other supplements I can use to promote cardiovascular health?

- What is the best heart-healthy diet for me: low-carb or low-fat?

- I am taking a statin; can I switch to a natural alternative?

- If I need a statin, what is the right dose for me?

- How can I avoid statin side effects? If side effects occur, what should I do?

- Cost is a factor for me: how can I get the treatment I need at the most affordable cost?

I am not categorically against statin medications. Statins help millions of people, especially those with documented heart disease. When taken by these people, statins reduce the risk of death from a heart attack by approximately 30 percent. This is an excellent result compared to other drugs, but it should be noted that the remaining 70 percent are not helped by taking a statin. The point is that while statins help millions of people, statins are not panaceas. Statins do not protect the majority of people who take them. Statins do not restore healthy arteries to the heart, brain, or peripheral circulatory system. Thus, if you are taking a statin drug, it is not a replacement for the many other things you can do to maintain or improve cardiovascular health.

NATURAL CHOLESTEROL-LOWERING REMEDIES

One of my concerns about statin drugs is that many doctors are prescribing super-strong statins to people with elevated cholesterol, but no history of heart disease or diabetes. I disagree with this aggressive, drug-first approach. For these people, statins should be the last, not first, choice.

Ten natural remedies have been shown to improve cholesterol levels (see Chapter 4), so you have many choices worth considering instead of statin drugs. These natural remedies only rarely cause side effects, and more often they provide "side benefits" that improve functioning in other systems of the body. Natural remedies are also much less expensive than prescription statins. These natural supplements are certainly worthy of consideration if you have elevated cholesterol, but are not high-risk for cardiovascular disease.

In addition, there are several other natural substances that do not lower cholesterol, but are needed by the human body to maintain cardiovascular health (see Chapter 5). Many people do not get adequate amounts of these nutrients in their diets, so you should consider supplementation with these natural substances whether or not you are taking a natural or prescription therapy to lower cholesterol.

Of course, the first therapy that any person with elevated cholesterol or other cardiovascular risk factors should adopt is a heart-healthy diet. This is not always easy, because different people can respond very differently to the same diet. Choosing the right diet based on your metabolism and genetics (as discussed in Chapter 6) is important for reducing cholesterol levels, and can do so by as much as with a moderate-strength statin.

THE PROBLEM OF STATIN SIDE EFFECTS

Side effects with statins are another reason to consider other options. Drug manufacturers claim that statins cause few side effects; the reality is that as many as 40 percent of statin users run into problems. One cardiologist recently wrote: "In many physicians' practices (including my own), muscle aches and weakness occur in approximately 30% of patients who take statins."[2] Serious memory problems also occur with statins. One doctor researching these problems stated: "We have people who have lost thinking ability so rapidly that within the course of a couple of months they went from being heads of major divisions of companies to not being able to balance a checkbook and being fired from their company."[3]

The Wall Street Journal reported:

> A number of critics believe drug companies have vastly understated side effects caused by statins — particularly muscle pains and memory problems. As a result, when patients complain of muscle aches and fuzzy thinking, many doctors do not even consider that a statin might be the culprit, and instead just assume the patient is getting old. Drug companies maintain that side effects are rare.[3]

The reality is that studies have shown that side effects occur much more frequently in everyday medical patients than is seen in drug studies.[4] With statins, the proof of the problem is that within a few years of starting on statins, 60 to 75 percent of patients discontinue treatment.[5,6] "Miracle" drugs cannot do much good if people cannot tolerate them.

If you need to take a statin medication, there are ways to do so while minimizing the risks of immediate and long-term side effects. This can be accomplished with precision prescribing, which is my term for individualizing treatment so that you get the right statin at the right dose for your individual goals and tolerance. Many people get side effects because their doctors prescribe statins at doses that are double or quadruple what people actually need. Doctors prescribe costly, super-strong statins such as Lipitor or Crestor when milder, safer statins will do.

In contrast, with individualized, precision prescribing, you will not get overmedicated. Lower, effective statin doses are tried first because lower doses are less likely to cause side effects. Yet, low-dose statins can be surprisingly effective, and you may never have to take a larger, riskier, costlier statin dosage. Space does not allow me to fully discuss this issue here, but if you or anyone you know is interested in how to take statin medication safely and inexpensively, please see my other book by Square One Publishers titled *What You Must Know About Statin Drugs and Their Natural Alternatives.*

ARE YOU SENSITIVE TO MEDICATIONS?

Some people are extremely sensitive to medications. If you are medication-sensitive, just a little medication goes a long way with you. Some statins are so strong, even the lowest dosage may still be too strong for you. You are not alone. Millions of people are medication-sensitive. These people frequently get side effects with medications and ultimately discontinue treatment. Doctors often ignore medication-sensitive patients or treat them like hypochondriacs, but medication sensitivities are real. Just as many people are sensitive to alcohol or coffee, many others are sensitive to powerful medications. If you are medication-sensitive, you will likely do better with a natural therapy for reducing cholesterol.

REDUCING CHOLESTEROL INEXPENSIVELY

More than $20 billion were spent on statin medications in America last year. The cost of statins and other expensive drugs not only drains the healthcare system of funds needed for other vital uses and drives up each of our insurance costs, but also forces many people to discontinue treatment that they need. Natural therapies are much less expensive than prescription statins, so natural therapies may not only be an effective and safe alternative for reducing cholesterol and improving cardiovascular health, but they may also allow you (and millions of other people) to continue treatment without interruption because of high costs.

Approximately 100 million Americans have elevated cholesterol. Most of these people do not need prescription drugs. A heart-healthy diet is sufficient for reducing cholesterol for many of these people, and a heart-healthy diet plus a natural supplement is sufficient for millions more. As you will see, the evidence is strong for natural therapies for reducing cholesterol or other elevated risk factors for cardiovascular disease. Scientific studies and clinical experience have established the effectiveness of these natural therapies. Although these natural therapies are available without a prescription, I advise people to work with a knowledgeable practitioner in deciding among the many choices of natural supplements, and in monitoring their effects on your levels of cholesterol or other risk factors.

LDL-C, HDL-C, C-Reactive Protein, Homocysteine, and Other Risk Factors for Heart Disease

Of all the common causes of premature death—heart attack, stroke, cancer, accidents, diabetes, and infectious diseases—the odds are greatest that you are going to die from a heart attack or stroke. This is true whether you are male or female.[1]

—Artemis Simopoulos, MD, former Chairman of the Nutrition Coordinating Committee at the National Institutes of Health

Each year, nearly 1 million Americans—over 2,500 a day, 100 an hour—die from cardiovascular disease, and 6 million are hospitalized. Each year, heart disease is our number one cause of death in men and women, and strokes are number three. Cardiovascular disease costs the American economy an estimated $274 billion annually. But this is not just an American problem: overall, about 45 percent of adults in Western societies die from cardiovascular disease.[2]

Most people are aware of the importance of maintaining cardiovascular health, but as more and more information emerges and the theories and guidelines keep changing, many people, including doctors, are confused. How can you prevent cardiovascular disease and maintain a healthy heart and blood vessels? How can you prevent a heart attack or stroke? What are the most important risk factors? What is the best approach? These are important questions, yet the answers keep changing as we identify new risk factors and redefine factors already recognized. It also depends on which expert you ask, especially on the issue of lowering cholesterol.

ABOUT CHOLESTEROL

Atherosclerosis underlies most cardiovascular disease. It is the development of plaques in arteries from accumulations of cholesterol combined with fatty droplets, platelets, and inflammatory cells. Atherosclerotic plaques can enlarge and block arteries to the heart, brain, kidneys, or limbs. Or the plaques can rupture, spewing their contents into arteries and triggering artery-blocking clots.

The body manufactures cholesterol for a reason. Cholesterol is an important component of healthy cells, and essential for normal body functioning. Cholesterol is needed for building cell membranes; for producing hormones such as estrogen, testosterone, and cortisol; and as a component of bile, which helps clear toxins from the body. But excess cholesterol can be a killer. An elevated cholesterol is defined as a cholesterol level of 240 mg/dl or above. A cholesterol level below 200 mg/dl is desirable, and a level between 200 and 239 mg/dl is borderline high. Since 1993, studies have repeatedly shown that lowering elevated cholesterol levels reduces coronary disease, heart attacks, and cardiac deaths.[3–7] That is why mainstream experts now recommend using statin drugs for 35 million Americans with elevated cholesterol levels.[8]

Most alternative doctors I know agree about the role of cholesterol in cardiovascular disease. "Your body is capable of producing all the cholesterol it needs, so there's no need to eat a lot of cholesterol," states Dr. Julian Whitaker, one of America's best known alternative physicians. "Excess cholesterol that isn't eliminated from your body is likely to be deposited in the walls of arteries, causing them to narrow and stiffen."[9] The result: cardiovascular mayhem—blocked arteries, heart attacks, strokes, reduced circulation to the kidneys and limbs.

LOW-DENSITY LIPOPROTEIN CHOLESTEROL (LDL-C)

Low-density lipoprotein cholesterol is often called the "bad cholesterol." Because cholesterol is not soluble, it must be transported in the bloodstream. This is accomplished by linking with protein-fat substances called lipoproteins. You are probably already familiar with LDL-C and HDL-C, the acronyms for low-density lipoprotein cholesterol and high-density lipoprotein cholesterol (see Table 2.1). Lowering cholesterol usually means lowering LDL-cholesterol, the bad low-density lipoprotein cholesterol that is closely linked with atherosclerosis. The highly respected National Cholesterol Education Program (Adult Treatment Panel III) (NCEP, for short) states:

Research from experimental animals, laboratory investigations, epidemiology, and genetic forms of hypercholesterolemia indicate that elevated LDL cholesterol is a major cause of coronary heart disease. In addition, recent clinical trials robustly show that LDL-lowering therapy reduces the risk for coronary heart disease.[10]

How important is it to reduce LDL-cholesterol? The risk of coronary disease is directly correlated with people's levels of LDL-C.[11] For example, people with coronary disease whose LDL-C levels are elevated have a twelve-fold greater likelihood of dying from a heart attack than people whose LDL-C levels are normal.[12] Reducing high LDL-C levels directly reduces cardiac risk. How much? The American Society of Hospital Pharmacists reports:

Table 2.1. Types of Cholesterol

TC = Total Cholesterol:
The total amount of cholesterol in the blood measured in mg/dl (milligrams per decaliter). Your total cholesterol level is comprised of HDL-C, LDL-C, and VLDL-C.

HDL-C = High-Density Lipoprotein Cholesterol:
The good cholesterol that protects against atherosclerosis. High HDL-C levels indicate a reduced risk of cardiovascular disease.

LDL-C = Low-Density Lipoprotein Cholesterol:
LDL-C is the bad cholesterol, linked to increased heart attacks, strokes, and sudden cardiac death. Lowering LDL-C reduces the risk. LDL-C is the key level in determining the type of treatment.

VLDL-C = Very Low-Density Lipoprotein Cholesterol:
Another type of bad cholesterol, usually present in much smaller amounts than LDL-C.

It has been estimated that each 1% reduction in LDL cholesterol may result in a 1% decrease in the incidence of coronary heart disease.[13]

These numbers are impressive, but they relate with the most accuracy to people with cardiovascular disease or serious risk factors. Moreover, LDL-C is not the whole story when it comes to predicting and preventing heart disease. Cardiologist William Davis writes:

> Cholesterol is nothing more than one of many risk factors for coronary heart disease, and just one of the contributors to the silent growth of plaque. Lowering cholesterol is still a good idea, but should be viewed in the proper perspective. Cholesterol does not reliably identify all people with hidden heart disease, nor does lowering it cure you of heart disease.[14]

In fact, according to Dr. Davis, for every 100 people with coronary heart disease, sixty or seventy will have a combination of two other risk factors, low levels of HDL-C and high levels of small particle LDL-C. In contrast, less than thirty of 100 people with coronary heart disease will have elevated LDL-C. Thus, it is important to know if you have a high level of LDL-C, and if so, how you can reduce it—but it is equally important to know about the other risk factors.

HIGH-DENSITY LIPOPROTEIN CHOLESTEROL (HDL-C)

HDL-cholesterol is often called the "good cholesterol" because HDL-C facilitates the transport of cholesterol in the bloodstream for elimination, leaving less cholesterol to accumulate in plaque. For this reason, a high level of HDL-C can offset some of the risk from a high LDL-C. The higher your HDL-C level, the lower your cardiac risk. Even if your LDL-C is very low (below 100 mg/dl), you still have a greater risk of heart disease if your HDL-C is low. Indeed, some studies suggest that HDL-C levels may be as important or even more important an indicator of cardiac risk than LDL-C. This appears to be especially true for women. Moreover, new studies using experimental drugs that enhance HDL-C have demonstrated the ability to partially reverse atherosclerosis.

Experts usually recommend an HDL-C level of at least 45 mg/dl for men and 55 mg/dl for women, but some consider an HDL-C of at least 60 mg/dl ideal. Some people have even higher HDL-C levels, but others have great difficulty reaching these levels because HDL-C levels are genetically determined to a large degree. Exercise and good oils (such as olive, canola) can elevate HDL-C levels modestly. Several natural therapies can be useful for raising HDL-C levels.

A low HDL-C is also seen in people with a condition known as "metabolic syndrome," which also includes elevated triglycerides, high blood pressure, and elevated glucose levels. Although people with metabolic syndrome have low LDL-C levels, they have an increased risk of developing heart disease and diabetes. People with metabolic syndrome often are overweight and may have elevated levels of C-reactive protein (see page 15). Metabolic syndrome is discussed further in Chapter 6.

UNDERSTANDING THE
CHOLESTEROL-TO-HDL-C RATIO

Sometimes it can get confusing when you try to assess the importance of your total cholesterol, LDL-C, and HDL-C levels together. For example, if your total cholesterol and LDL-C are elevated, but so is your HDL-C, how do these balance out? Is your overall risk high or low? A shorthand way of answering this question is with the use of the cholesterol-to-HDL-C ratio. If you divide your total cholesterol by your HDL-C, you will obtain a number. For example, if your total cholesterol is 200 mg/dl and your HDL-C is 50, your cholesterol-to-HDL-C ratio is 4 (or precisely, 4:1). A cholesterol-to-HDL-C ratio above 5 is considered high risk; a ratio of 3.5 or lower is considered optimal; a ratio in between is considered lower risk.

The cholesterol-to-HDL-C ratio is a handy way to assess your risk, but it can be misleading. A ratio of 4 may be perfectly acceptable if you are healthy and have few risk factors for cardiovascular disease. In contrast, if you have severe coronary artery disease or diabetes, a cholesterol-to-HDL-C ratio of 4 may be too high. You would want an LDL-C below 100 or even 70 mg/dl, and an HDL-C of at least 50, preferably 60 mg/dl. This would produce a cholesterol-to-HDL-C ratio of 2 or less. In other words, your cholesterol-to-HDL-C ratio must be evaluated in the context of your situation. This is explained at greater length in Chapter 3, which will explain how to identify your risk category and determine whether you require a reduction of LDL-C.

C-REACTIVE PROTEIN:
THE IMPORTANT NEW RISK FACTOR

Thousands of cardiac deaths each year occur in people with normal cholesterol levels. Clearly, other factors are involved. New studies suggest that an elevated level of C-reactive protein (CRP), an indicator of inflammation, may be as important an indicator of cardiac risk as cholesterol levels.[15,16] In fact, emerging evidence suggests that an elevated CRP may also be an indicator of an increased risk of high blood pressure, colon cancer, Alzheimer's disease, and perhaps many other disorders.

C-reactive protein is produced in the liver and other tissues in response to infection or inflammation anywhere in the body. CRP is manufactured as part of the body's immune response against infection and injury, but this immune response can cause damage if it produces excess inflammation in a person's own tissues. For years, experts have suspected that inflammation in artery walls played an important role in causing atherosclerosis—and in other diseases, too. "Forward-thinking cardiologists now suspect that internal inflammation is the root cause of many diseases including those of the heart and blood vessels," states cardiologist Stephen Sinatra.[17]

It is now believed that millions of Americans with elevated CRP (also known as "high-sensitivity CRP") are at risk, even though their cholesterol levels are normal. Dr. Paul Ridker, Director of the Center for Cardiovascular Disease Prevention at Brigham and Women's Hospital in Boston, told *The New York Times*, "From 25 to 30 million healthy, middle-aged Americans are at far higher risk than they and their doctors understand them to be, because we're not taking inflammatory factors into account."[18]

Indeed, some doctors believe that CRP is a more accurate indicator of cardiovascular risk than LDL-C, especially in women.[15] Dr. Sinatra states:

> C-reactive protein (CRP) may be the most predictive for cardiovascular killers such as heart attack, stroke, and vascular disease. Studies have shown that people with elevated CRP run two times the risk of dying from a cardiovascular-related problem compared with those who have high cholesterol levels. Combine a cholesterol burden with a markedly elevated CRP and your risk of heart attack and stroke increases by a factor of nine.[17]

While research continues on defining the actual importance of CRP as an indicator of cardiovascular risk, some experts believe that inflammation, as reflected by CRP, has always been the major factor underlying atherosclerosis. Dr. Uffe Ravnskov and others have written extensively about the holes in the cholesterol theory, and that mainstream medicine's obsession with reducing cholesterol levels has always been misguided.[19]

The American Heart Association and the U.S. Centers for Disease Control and Prevention now recommend CRP tests for people at risk for cardiovascular disease. A CRP level below 1 is low risk; 1–3, moderate risk; above 3, high risk. Some doctors are already ordering CRP tests on all patients and prescribing statin drugs to everyone with an elevated level of CRP, yet many experts believe that prescribing drugs is premature. "Before we have tens of millions of Americans placed on statins because of their CRP, we need randomized clinical trials to show they would benefit," Dr. Sidney Smith, professor of medicine at University of North Carolina at Chapel Hill and chief science officer at the American Heart Association, told *The Wall Street Journal*.[20]

CRP levels are improved by the same factors that improve cardiovascular health: exercise, good diet, maintaining a healthy weight, not smoking. Women should be aware that the hormonal therapy for menopausal symptoms might raise their CRP level considerably.[21] Aspirin appears to be effective for reducing CRP, probably due to its anti-inflammatory effect. But the big push today for treating elevated CRP is with statins. However, before rushing to prescribed drugs for elevated CRP, shouldn't we be asking why CRP levels are elevated in the first place?

One possibility is that our diets are deficient in nutrients needed by humans to maintain a healthy balance between pro-inflammatory and anti-inflammatory systems. One important nutrient for maintaining anti-inflammatory effect is omega-3 oils from fish and whole foods. The Western diet is terribly deficient in omega-3 oils. Meanwhile, Westerners get huge amounts of omega-6 oils (safflower, sunflower, corn, soy, peanut oils) that have a pro-inflammatory effect. Could it be that we are seeing higher incidences of many types of inflammatory disorders like rheumatoid arthritis, lupus, Crohn's disease—and markers like elevated CRP—because our diets are skewed toward pro-inflammatory nutrients?

The proper balance between omega-6 (O6) and omega-3 (O3) oils in the human diet should be 2:1 or even 1:1. In the U.S., it is 17:1. With people eating so many pro-inflammatory oils decade after decade, is it really surprising that we are seeing a tide of inflammatory disorders today? In comparison, in Greece the O6/O3 ratio is 2:1, and the incidence of cardiovascular disease is much lower.[22,23] For more on the many benefits of omega-3 oils, see Chapter 5.

Although many doctors immediately prescribe statin drugs to patients with elevated CRP, there are many reasons to pause before reaching for the prescription pad. We are just learning about this indicator and what influences it. For example, a study in the *Journal of the American College of Nutrition* demonstrated that 515 mg/day of vitamin C reduced CRP 24 percent.[24] Might vitamin C alone, or combined with fish oils or other natural substances, reduce CRP as much as statins? It would be much cheaper, safer, and physiologically beneficial to the body. These and many other questions await further study.

OTHER RISK FACTORS

As if it isn't already complicated enough, several other factors have now been linked with an increased risk of atherosclerosis, heart attacks and strokes, and premature cardiovascular death.

Triglycerides

Although not a type of cholesterol, triglycerides, like cholesterol, are common fats in the body. Elevated blood levels of triglycerides are directly linked to heart attacks and strokes, and the risk is magnified if you also have a high LDL-C, low HDL-C, or a preponderance of small, dense LDL-C particles. Your fasting triglyceride level should be below 150 mg/dl. A borderline triglyceride level is 150–199; elevated, 200–499; extremely high, over 500 mg/dl.

High carbohydrate diets and alcohol can exacerbate triglyceride problems, so treatment includes reducing consumption of simple carbohydrates (healthful vegetables are okay) and alcohol, as well as weight loss and smoking cessation in people who are overweight or smokers. Statins are sometimes prescribed for reducing triglyceride levels, but natural niacin therapies are often more effective. Omega-3 oils also reduce triglycerides.

Small Particle LDL-Cholesterol

Small particle LDL-cholesterol is a newly recognized risk factor for heart disease. LDL-C particles in the bloodstream come in various sizes. The body can metabolize large particles quickly, but small, dense LDL-C particles can attach to atherosclerotic plaques, increasing plaque size. Indeed, new studies suggest that longevity may be linked more closely to having large LDL-C and HDL-C particles, rather than low levels of LDL-C. Testing for LDL-C particle size is not routinely done, but it may be useful if you have a family history of heart disease, because the tendency toward small particle LDL-C is usually genetically determined. Small particle LDL-C is worsened by a high-carbohydrate/low-fat diet, if it raises your triglyceride level. Simple carbs are the main culprit and should be avoided (see Chapter 6). Weight loss and exercise can help reduce small-particle LDL-C levels. Niacin therapies are the most effective pill treatment (see Chapter 4).

Lipoprotein A

Lipoprotein A consists of a molecule of LDL linked with a protein (apoprotein A). An elevated level of lipoprotein A is a major risk factor for coronary artery disease. Some practitioners believe it may be the most important single risk factor in assessing cardiovascular risk. An elevated lipoprotein A is usually genetically determined and found in about 20 percent of the population. Most doctors do not routinely screen for elevated lipoprotein A, but testing for this factor should be considered for at-risk individuals or those with family histories of heart disease or stroke. Recent reports also suggest that lipoprotein A is a major risk factor in older people.[25,26]

Mainstream medical dogma states that diet and weight loss do not affect lipoprotein A levels very much, but some alternative practitioners report significant lipoprotein A reductions with strict elimination diets.[27] Niacin appears to be the only reliable treatment for reducing lipoprotein A levels. Statin drugs do not usually improve lipoprotein A levels significantly. Indeed, a recent anecdotal report suggests that statin drugs may increase lipoprotein A levels in some people.[27]

Homocysteine

An elevated homocysteine level is linked not only to coronary artery disease and congestive heart failure, but also to impaired cognitive functioning and Parkinson's and Alzheimer's diseases in the elderly, pregnancy complications, birth defects, increased death rates in diabetics, and possibly cancer. Elevated homocysteine levels may indicate abnormal functioning of the inner lining of blood vessels (the endothelium) and, possibly, an increased tendency for clotting. People with elevated homocysteine levels have much greater risks of having heart attacks or dying of heart disease than people with normal homocysteine levels. As many as 20 percent of people with heart disease and 30 percent of people with other cardiovascular diseases have high values of homocysteine.

Homocysteine accrues in harmful amounts in people who are unable to metabolize the amino acid methionine. Methionine is abundant in meat, so reducing meat intake lowers homocysteine levels in these people. Dr. Kilmer S. McCully, who discovered the homocysteine-artery disease link in 1969, believes that atherosclerosis is primarily a disease of protein metabolism from the excess protein in Western diets.[28] According to McCully, limiting animal protein, caffeine, and alcohol, and performing exercise and stress reduction, can reduce homocysteine levels substantially.

If your homocysteine test was drawn while you had an acute infection such as the flu, it might be temporarily elevated and should be retested after the illness has ended. Folic acid, in combination with vitamins B_6 and B_{12}, is usually effective in facilitating the body's metabolism and utilization of methionine, thereby reducing homocysteine levels. Sometimes megadoses of folic acid are required. When folic acid does not work, another alternative product, trimethylglycine (TMG), often does. On the other hand, niacin can raise homocysteine levels in some people, so your homocysteine level should be checked if you take any form of niacin. For guidelines about healthy homocysteine levels and the use of folic acid, see Chapter 5.

Fibrinogen

An elevated level of fibrinogen is linked to an increased risk of strokes, heart attacks, and cardiovascular death. Fibrinogen is a blood protein involved in the normal process of clotting, but elevated levels of fibrinogen can make platelets stick more readily to atherosclerotic plaques and form clots when these plaques rupture. Elevated levels of fibrinogen may also indicate a tendency toward atherosclerosis, dysfunction of the vascular lining (the endothelium), and other types of vascular disease. Elevated fibrinogen levels are more predictive of cardiovascular risk for women than for men. Mainstream doctors and some alternative doctors recommend aspirin (81 mg daily) to reduce platelet clumping and clotting in at-risk patients, because studies have proven that aspirin can reduce these patients' risk of heart attacks and atherosclerotic strokes. Other alternative doctors recommend natural therapies with anticlotting effects such as omega-3 fatty acids (fish oils), garlic, arginine, bromelain, vitamin E, or tumeric or curcumin (a tumeric extract).

WHAT YOU SHOULD DO

All of the risk factors discussed in this chapter are important. Although experts may debate the relative importance of high LDL-C and low HDL-C, there is little debate that elevated levels of C-reactive protein, homocysteine, small particle LDL-C, fibrinogen, and lipoprotein A are clear risk factors for cardiovascular disease, and they should be rectified. Other risk factors include obesity, stress, smoking, and physical inactivity.

What if your cholesterol levels are not elevated, but you have a strong family history of coronary artery disease or cardiac death at an early age? You should have all of the other risk factors measured. Tests for triglycerides, CRP, homocysteine, and fibrinogen levels can usually be done at the same time you get cholesterol levels measured. In addition, many mainstream laboratories are now offering the VAP (Vertical Auto Profile) analysis, an in-depth analysis of more than a dozen cardiovascular risk factors including subtypes of LDL-C and HDL-C, as well as lipoprotein A and small particle LDL-C. The VAP analysis identifies twice as many people at risk than routine cholesterol tests. Most likely, one or more of these risk factors will be elevated, and you should have it treated.

What should you do if you have elevated cholesterol or LDL-C? This is the key question, and I will answer it in the next chapter.

Is Your Cholesterol Level Too High? And If So, What To Do About It

There is a great deal of confusion today among consumers, and even some doctors, about how to define elevated cholesterol levels and how to treat people with them. I have heard many stories of people placed on statin drugs when their cholesterol numbers did not warrant drug therapy. On the other hand, surveys have shown that many people who do need cholesterol reduction are not receiving any kind of nutritional counseling, or natural or drug therapy. When statin drugs are prescribed, the dosages are sometimes too strong and cause unnecessary side effects. Other times the dosages are too mild to accomplish the goal. This chapter will explain how you can determine if your cholesterol levels are elevated, and the following chapter will offer a variety of natural therapies for reducing elevated cholesterol and LDL-C.

THE IMPORTANCE OF DEFINING YOUR LDL-C GOAL

Recently, while I was appearing on a radio show, a woman called in and asked, "Do I need Lipitor? My doctor wants me to start taking 20 mg of Lipitor, but I disagree." The woman was forty-six years old and had no heart disease or major risk factors. Her cholesterol numbers were: total cholesterol, 240; LDL-C, 100; HDL-C, 110 mg/dl.

A cholesterol level of 240 is considered high. Most of the 42 million Americans with cholesterol this high or higher need cholesterol reduction, but this woman did not. If you look at the current American Heart Association guidelines on page 30, you can see that this woman was in the low risk category. Moreover, a large part of her elevated total cholesterol was from her HDL-C of 110, which is highly protective against heart disease. Her ratio of LDL-C to HDL-C was less than 1, an excellent ratio. So why did her doctor recommend a strong dosage of a very strong statin drug?

This is one of the problems with the drug-first mentality of today. Some doctors are so overly enthusiastic about statin drugs, they are prescribing strong statin drugs for people who require mild treatment or no treatment at all. Recent studies conducted by drug companies have shown that lowering LDL-C to below 70 mg/dl reduces heart attacks and cardiac deaths in people with severe coronary artery disease. This is important information if you have coronary artery disease, but some doctors have misinterpreted these studies and are applying the goal of an LDL-C below 70 mg/dl to everyone. There is absolutely no basis for this. For people without coronary artery disease or diabetes, the American Heart Association guidelines remain the same. For the woman mentioned above, her goal was an LDL-C below 160 mg/dl. Her LDL was already way below this.

Some experts believe that the LDL-C goals in these guidelines should be lower. Sooner or later, the American Heart Association may adopt some of these lower guidelines, so I also include these lower levels of LDL-C on pages 30–31. For example, for people in the low-risk category, the current guideline is an LDL-C below 160, but some experts suggest an LDL-C below 130. For people in the moderate-risk categories, the current guideline is an LDL-C below 130, but some experts recommend an LDL-C below 100.

Many people can achieve these LDL-C goals with a heart-healthy diet and natural cholesterol-lowering therapies. Too often, unfortunately, doctors turn first to statin drugs, often at excessive doses. More is not necessarily better with statin drugs. The stronger the statin therapy, the greater the risks. Statins often cause muscle aches, joint pain, fatigue, memory impairment, thinking impairment, abdominal discomfort, and liver injury. Sometimes these reactions are severe, and, rarely, deaths have been reported from muscle breakdown, kidney failure, and liver toxicity. All of these side effects are dose-related: the higher the dosage, the greater the risk. In addition, some people have developed nerve injuries from years of taking statin drugs, and the higher the dosage, the greater the risk.

HOW YOU CAN GET THE RIGHT TREATMENT FOR THE RIGHT GOAL

To attain your treatment goals, to minimize the risks of any treatment, and to minimize your costs, you need to determine your LDL-C goals—and you need to ensure that your doctor does the same. Today, it appears that many doctors simply prescribe the strongest statin drugs (Lipitor, Zocor, Crestor) at the strong dosages that are intensively advertised and constantly pushed by the pharmaceutical sales reps who visit doctors' offices. If you have not done your homework, you may receive a statin drug or dosage that is inappropriate and places you at unnecessary risk.

People tell me, "If my doctor recommends a statin, what can I do? I don't know enough to question the decision. The doctor knows much more than I do and is only trying to help me. I feel uninformed. I feel that I have to accept the doctor's opinion. What else can I do?"

There is a lot you can do. First, have your blood tested for total cholesterol, LDL-C, HDL-C, and triglycerides. Many people already have this information or can get it from their doctor's office.

Second, from the chart on page 30, determine your risk category: is it low, moderate, moderate-high, or high? People with heart disease or diabetes are automatically in the high-risk category. The other categories are based on other risk factors, such as whether you have high blood pressure, a family history of early coronary artery disease, an HDL-C below 40, or smoke cigarettes. The vast majority of people with elevated LDL-C fit into the low- or moderate-risk groups.

Third, compare your LDL-C level with the LDL-C level recommended for your risk category. If your LDL-C is above the recommended level, calculate how much LDL-C reduction you will need to reach the recommended level. For example, if you are in the low-risk category and your LDL-C is 180 mg/dl, you want to reduce your LDL-C to below 160. This is a reduction of at least 21 mg/dl, or about 12 percent. This can be accomplished with the right heart-healthy diet or with natural therapies.

Another example. If you are in the moderate-risk category and your LDL-C is 140 mg/dl, you want to reduce it by at least 11 mg/dl to the American Heart Association goal of below 130 mg/dl. However, your doctor may prefer a goal of 100 mg/dl. This will require a reduction of at least 40 mg/dl, or about 30 percent. A heart-healthy diet plus natural therapies can accomplish this. A statin is unnecessary.

Most important, if you have done your homework, you now can be an active participant in discussions with your doctor about these issues. You will know your cholesterol levels and understand what each one means. You will know your treatment category based on the American Heart Association guidelines. You will know your LDL-C and HDL-C goals, and you will know if you require improvement in any of these categories. And you will also know about natural alternatives that can be used before turning to statin drugs. In fact, you will know a lot more that many doctors.

THE HIGH-RISK GROUP

If you are in the high-risk category, you likely have coronary artery disease or another type of atherosclerotic vascular disease, or diabetes, which frequently leads to vascular disease, or other serious risk factors. Your cholesterol goal is an LDL-C below 100 mg/dl. Some experts are now recommending an LDL-C below 70 mg/dl for people in the high-risk category.

If you already have coronary or atherosclerotic disease, you may also have heard the term "secondary prevention." Secondary prevention refers to people who already have cardiovascular disease, and for whom the goal of cholesterol-lowering therapy is to prevent further damage. In contrast, "primary prevention" refers to people without vascular disease, and the goal of cholesterol-lowering therapy is to prevent the development of coronary or other atherosclerotic disease.

Treatment that can prevent further damage is imperative for people in the high-risk group. For example, mortality is high for people who survive a first heart attack but do not receive ongoing treatment: 5 percent mortality a year with a cumulative cardiovascular mortality of 70 percent after fifteen years. After a second heart attack, cardiovascular mortality is 10 percent per year without consistent treatment.[1] "The high mortality rate emphasizes the need to ensure that everyone who has had a myocardial infarction (heart attack), even years previously, receives effective preventive treatment," stated an article in the *Archives of Internal Medicine*.[2]

This is why many experts are now recommending an LDL-C below 70 mg/dl for high-risk patients. Some people may be able to reach this goal with natural approaches, but statin treatment is often needed. In Chapter 7, I will explain when and how to use statin drugs safely and effectively.

Now that you have determined your risk category and how much LDL-C reduction you need, you may find that you can reach your treatment goal with one of the many natural therapies that are presented in the next chapter.

Defining Your Risk Category and LDL-C Lowering Requirement

There are four risk categories: low, moderate, moderate-high, and high risk. In order to find your category, you need to determine how many risk factors you have. Risk factors include (add 1 risk factor for each that you have): Age (males over 44, females over 54); high blood pressure (even if being treated); cigarette smoking; a family history of early coronary disease; an HDL level below 40 mg/dl. If your HDL level is 60 or higher, you can subtract one risk factor.

Low-Risk Category: You are in this category if you have 0 or 1 risk factor and do not have cardiovascular disease or diabetes. Your goal is an LDL-C level below 160 mg/dl (some experts recommend an LDL-C below 130).

If your LDL-C is between 160 to 189: you should initiate diet and other lifestyle changes.*

If your LDL-C is 190 or higher: you should initiate diet and other lifestyle changes. If these do not reduce your LDL-C below 160, a cholesterol-lowering therapy should be considered.

Moderate-Risk Category: You are in this category if you have 2 or more risk factors, but you do not have cardiovascular disease or diabetes, and other risk indicators are few.** Your goal is an LDL-C level below 130 mg/dl (some experts recommend an LDL-C below 100).

If your LDL-C is 130 to 159: you should initiate diet and other lifestyle changes.*

If your LDL-C is 160 or higher: you should initiate diet and other lifestyle changes. If these do not reduce your LDL-C below 130, a cholesterol-lowering therapy should be considered.

Moderate-High-Risk Category: You are in this category if you do not have cardiovascular disease or diabetes, but you have 2 or more risk factors and your other risk indicators are considerable.** Your goal is an LDL-C level below 130 mg/dl (many experts now recommend an LDL-C below 100).

If your LDL-C is 130 or higher: initiate diet and other lifestyle changes.* If these do not reduce your LDL-C below 130 (or below 100, if this is your goal), a cholesterol-lowering therapy should be considered.

No matter what your LDL-C level is, you should initiate diet and other lifestyle changes if: you are overweight by 20 pounds or more; you are physically inactive; you have an elevated triglyceride level; your HDL-C is below 40; or you have metabolic syndrome (see Chapter 6).

High-Risk Category: You are in the high-risk category if you have heart or other atherosclerotic vascular disease, or diabetes, or other factors that indicate a very high degree of risk.** The goal for this category is an LDL-C below 100 mg/dl. However, for people with advanced cardiovascular disease or diabetes, or who are otherwise considered at very high risk, an LDL-C below 70 mg/dl is preferable.

If your LDL-C is 100 or higher (or above 70 if this is your goal): you should initiate diet and other lifestyle changes as well as cholesterol-lowering therapy.

No matter what your LDL-C level is, you should initiate diet and other lifestyle changes if: you are overweight by 20 pounds or more; you are physically inactive; you have an elevated triglyceride level; your HDL-C is below 40; or you have metabolic syndrome (see Chapter 6).

*Lifestyle changes include regular moderate exercise, maintaining a healthy weight, not smoking, and stress reduction. Initiating dietary and other lifestyle changes are very important because they can reduce your cardiovascular risk via several mechanisms, in addition to lowering your LDL-C.

**Other risk indicators: The measurement of cardiovascular risk sometimes involves a second, complicated calculation that assesses additional risk factors. The best way to obtain this calculation is via the American Heart Association's program at: http://www.americanheart.org/presenter.jhtml?identifier=3003499.

This information is adapted from the 2004 guidelines from the National Cholesterol Education Program.[3]

TEN ALTERNATIVE THERAPIES FOR LOWERING CHOLESTEROL AND OTHER RISK FACTORS

In an optimal healthcare system, solutions for many disorders would begin with nutrition, then natural interventions, then pharmaceuticals. This is not the predominant model today, yet natural therapies have gained an unprecedented role in many people's healthcare. In 2000, 150 million Americans spent $17 billion on dietary supplements. The establishment has still not come to grips with this. In 2002, the U.S. Department of Health and Human Services reported that "most complementary and alternative modalities have not yet been scientifically studied and found to be safe and effective."[1] The American Medical Association added: "There is little evidence to confirm the safety or efficacy of most alternative therapies."[2]

These attitudes miss the point. First, there are many alternative therapies that have now been proven in studies. Second, people do not like taking prescription drugs with their side effects and exorbitant costs. Millions of people are turned off by the high-pressure marketing of the drug industry and the "drug-first" mentality of many doctors. Perhaps most important, people instinctively understand the potential benefits of using natural alternatives that are more physiologic and safer than prescription drugs.

Today, there are several natural remedies that are proven to reduce LDL-C, and a few that raise the good HDL-C. However, because of the limited financial resources of their manufacturers and little interest among mainstream doctors and journals, studies on these natural products are far fewer than on prescription statins. Nutriceutical manufacturers cannot match the billions in annual profits of the drug companies, so placebo-controlled, double-blind studies of natural therapies are few, and there are hardly any long-term studies of these products' impact on morbidity and mortality. Still, the studies that exist are promising, and clinical experience has often been rewarding.

Dr. Robert Rowen, a practitioner of integrative medicine in Santa Rosa, CA, board certified in family practice and a fellow of the American Academy of Family Physicians, wrote to me:

> Regarding alternatives to statins, my brother is a good case in point. With a cholesterol of 230, his doctor tried to talk him into taking a statin. Instead, I recommended a standard dose of red yeast rice and guggulipid. His LDL-cholesterol dropped 30 points. I rarely have to use statin drugs between red yeast, guggulipid, niacin, and dietary change. The only time statins may be useful is for familial hypercholesterolemia [a severe, genetic form of elevated cholesterol]. I have not written an original prescription for statin drugs EVER.

Dr. Rowen is not alone. Thousands of doctors in

North and South America, Europe, and Asia use alternative therapies to lower cholesterol without resorting to prescription drugs. These methods may not be FDA approved, but this does not mean they do not work. Doctors use prescription drugs everyday in ways that are not FDA approved, so there is nothing unusual about choosing a proven-effective natural alternative for lowering cholesterol or CRP.

Some doctors are uncomfortable using natural alternatives because it means making decisions on less scientific data than with prescription drugs. But following patients' cholesterol and CRP levels can gauge the effectiveness of a natural alternative. For patients with moderate cholesterol or CRP elevations, the situation is not an emergency, so there's time to try natural, less expensive methods if this is what the patient desires. Medical science supports decisions by doctors that involve trying unorthodox, yet reasonable, methods in situations that warrant them. Using natural supplements is a valid approach for you if your cholesterol and CRP levels are monitored.

RED YEAST RICE

> *Chinese red yeast rice has significant potential to reduce healthcare costs and contribute to public health by reducing heart disease risk in individuals with moderate elevations of circulating cholesterol levels.*[3]
> —JOURNAL OF ALTERNATIVE AND COMPLEMENTARY MEDICINE

This viewpoint is also reflected in the *Journal of the American Academy of Family Physicians*, which usually takes a very cautious approach regarding natural supplements.

But it did not hesitate to publish a study of red yeast rice for reducing cholesterol. The conclusion: "So far, red yeast rice has proved to be a cost-saving lipid-lowering medication."[4] Red yeast rice has been used in China since 800 A.D. It is produced by fermenting rice with a yeast (*Monascus Purpurus*) that gives it a reddish hue. Red yeast rice contains approximately ten compounds that are similar in action to prescription statins, particularly lovastatin, the statin in Mevacor. Thus, for doctors who are adamant about obtaining statin-like effects, red yeast rice is a good alternative.

Yet, some doctors are not impressed. One told me, "I look at it as a watered-down version of Mevacor, so I don't use it." If he wants a statin-like effect, he said, he prescribes a statin, because the studies of effectiveness are far more extensive and the production of statins, regulated by the FDA, is guaranteed to deliver a standardized amount in each pill.

On the other hand, red yeast rice does not seem to cause the typical side effects—muscle pain, abdominal discomfort, liver irritation—that commonly occur with statins. In addition, red yeast rice also acts as an antioxidant and may prevent the oxidation of cholesterol in the bloodstream. Dr. Allan Magaziner, an alternative practitioner in Cherry Hill, NJ, and president of the American College for the Advancement of Medicine (ACAM), explains,

> I have used red yeast rice in more than five hundred patients, and it is remarkably effective. It is also very well tolerated. No muscle aches or pains. No liver enzyme elevations. It doesn't appear to lower coenzyme Q_{10} levels, although I have patients take a little

CoQ_{10} for safety anyway. Red yeast rice does contain statin-like compounds, but I suspect that because it contains small amounts of multiple compounds, no one of them is large enough to produce problems.

Dr. Magaziner uses red yeast rice for people with moderate cholesterol elevations in the 200–260 range. He obtains LDL-C reductions of 20 percent to 25 percent and small increases in HDL-C. Some people get even better results. "I've seen some great results that are usually apparent within two months, sometimes within weeks," Dr. Magaziner told me. "Red yeast rice is my first choice for lowering cholesterol levels."

The usual dose of red yeast rice is 1200 mg twice daily. According to Dr. David Heber, a nutrition expert at UCLA and author of *What Color Is Your Diet*, a daily dose of red yeast rice contains about 5 mg of lovastatin. Dr. Magaziner sometimes starts with 1200 mg once daily, and then increases the dose if necessary. In recalcitrant cases, he adds policosanol. Scientific studies support Dr. Magaziner's findings. Studies in China demonstrated cholesterol reductions of 11 percent to 32 percent with red yeast rice. American studies derived similar results:

- *American Journal of Clinical Nutrition:* In a double-blind, placebo-controlled study of 83 subjects, ages 34–78, with total cholesterol levels of 204–338 and LDL-C levels of 128–277, 1200 mg twice daily of red yeast rice reduced LDL-C 22 percent on average, significantly better than placebo. No significant side effects occurred. The authors commented: "Red yeast rice significantly reduces total cholesterol, LDL cholesterol, and total triglyceride concentrations compared with placebo and provides a new, novel, food-based approach to lowering cholesterol in the general population."[5]

- *Nutrition:* In a small, placebo-controlled, double-blind study of AIDS patients with elevated cholesterol, 1200 mg of red yeast rice twice daily reduced LDL-C 32 percent on average. No side effects occurred.[6]

An additional benefit of red yeast rice is that, like prescription statins, it may reduce elevated C-reactive protein levels. Many alternative doctors prefer to treat elevated CRP with exercise, omega-3 oils, vitamin C and/or vitamin E, which work sometimes. When these do not reduce CRP enough, a statin—prescription statins or red yeast rice—may be useful.

Although red yeast rice is available over the counter, it should be used with medical supervision. Red yeast rice has been used in America for more than a decade, but at times it was difficult to obtain, so it has not been used extensively here. So far, its track record appears good. Reported side effects are few (headaches, muscle or stomach pain). Liver and kidney effects have not been seen in human studies, but liver enzymes should be checked anyway.[7] Red yeast rice should not be used during pregnancy or with drugs that are contraindicated with statin medications.

Red yeast rice also provides an alternative for people who need, but cannot afford, prescription statins. Based on my own brief survey of pharmacies a few years ago, statins cost from $85 to $120 per month, whereas red yeast rice costs only $20 to $30 per month. Red yeast rice is not FDA approved for reducing cholesterol or treating cardiovascular disease.

INTERMEDIATE-ACTING NIACIN

Niacin (nicotinic acid) is the rare therapy recommended by both mainstream and alternative doctors. Niacin was the first therapy proven to improve cholesterol levels. At doses much higher than the recommended daily allowance, niacin reduces total cholesterol and LDL-C, while raising HDL-C. I agree with this statement in a recent consumer health newsletter: "Niacin is the most potent pill you can take to raise your HDL ('good') cholesterol."[8] For example, Niaspan, a prescription niacin preparation, can reduce LDL-C 5 percent to 25 percent, triglycerides 20 percent to 50 percent, and increase HDL-C 15 percent to 35 percent.[9]

Niacin is vitamin B_3, which is necessary for processing carbohydrates into energy or fat. Niacin also plays a role in the metabolism of cholesterol. Another form of vitamin B_3, niacinamide, has no effects on cholesterol metabolism. Niacin not only has favorable effects on cholesterol levels, but also on triglyceride and fibrinogen levels. It also reduces levels of small-particle LDL-C and lipoprotein A, which some doctors believe are more important risk indicators than an elevated LDL-C. Most importantly, niacin has been shown to reduce people's risk of heart attacks, including the risk of recurrent heart attacks in cardiac patients, as well as overall mortality. As a result of niacin's beneficial effects, some practitioners use it as a first-line therapy for cardiac risk factors. Dr. Julian Whitaker states, "Niacin has been around for a long time as a cholesterol-lowering agent, and is the best single remedy for lowering LDL cholesterol and raising HDL."[10] Other doctors prefer using niacin as a second-line treatment or combined with other therapies. Because 25 percent to 50 percent of high-risk coronary patients do not reach their LDL-C goals even with the strongest statin doses, niacin is often added.[11] However, niacin should be used cautiously in conjunction with statin drugs or red yeast rice, with the direction of a healthcare practitioner.

Niacin may sometimes increase homocysteine levels. For a long time, niacin was thought to also increase blood glucose levels, but this does not seem to be the case for most people. However, if you take any form of niacin, your fasting serum glucose and homocysteine levels should be measured when your cholesterol levels are checked. Because niacin can raise uric acid levels or activate peptic ulcers, it is usually avoided in people with histories of gout or ulcers. Niacin is usually contraindicated if you have liver disease or consume substantial quantities of alcohol. All niacin products should be used cautiously with blood thinners.

Doctors generally do not recommend plain niacin because it is very short acting and frequently causes flushing, itching, headaches, and stomach pain. At the doses needed to benefit cholesterol levels, flushing can be intense and causes many people to quit treatment. These problems have led to the development of slowly absorbed, long-acting niacin products. However, some early sustained-release preparations caused liver toxicity, so intermediate-release (or "extended-release") niacin preparations, with better side-effect profiles, have become the preferred approach. These include prescription preparations such as Niaspan and over-the-counter Endur-acin and inositol hexaniacinate.

Prescription Niacin: Niaspan

Niaspan is the preferred intermediate-acting niacin preparation among many mainstream doctors. Niaspan is FDA approved and listed in the PDR, yet it does have some adverse effects. Flushing, warmth, redness, and itching are less than with plain niacin, but still commonly occur. The manufacturer informs patients that taking aspirin or an anti-inflammatory drug such as ibuprofen thirty minutes before taking Niaspan may minimize flushing. Other adverse effects include headache, sweating, dizziness, nausea, heartburn, diarrhea, and palpitations.[12,13] Niaspan causes liver enzyme elevations in about 1 percent of patients, and a reversible form of hepatitis can occur. Because Niaspan side effects are dose-related, as are most side effects of niacin preparations, doctors usually initiate Niaspan therapy at 500 mg, then increase gradually to 1,000–2,000 mg/day. Women often respond to lower Niaspan doses than men. Liver enzyme levels should be checked regularly. Niaspan is a prescription drug and expensive.

Over-the-Counter Endur-acin

A well-known brand of over-the-counter extended-acting niacin is Endur-acin. Endur-acin is similar to Niaspan in that it contains niacin, which enters the body gradually from a sustained-release formulation. Endur-acin can cause side effects similar to those listed above for Niaspan. Flushing can be reduced by taking Endur-acin with meals or taking one 325 mg tablet of aspirin. Endur-acin is used at lower dosages than the other niacin compounds discussed in this chapter. The recommended initial dosage of Endur-acin is 250 mg/day, which may be increased gradually to 1,000–2,000 mg/day in divided doses. The manufacturer advises supervision by a doctor for the use of doses above 500 mg/day. Liver enzyme levels should be checked regularly. Endur-acin is much less expensive than Niaspan.

Over-the-Counter Inositol Hexaniacinate (Hexanicotinate, Nicotinate)

Many alternative doctors prefer a different type niacin derivative: inositol hexaniacinate. Inositol hexaniacinate is available over the counter and is much less expensive than Niaspan. Inositol hexaniacinate appears to cause considerably fewer side effects:

- *Alternative Medicine Review:* "The need for a safer approach to niacin supplementation has resulted in the investigation of niacin esters. One of the most widely studied of these is inositol hexaniacinate. In numerous trials it has been found virtually free of the side effects associated with conventional niacin therapy. Extensive research has found inositol hexaniacinate to be effective in the treatment of hyperlipidemia, Raynaud's disease and intermittent claudication."[14]

- *Nutrition Action Health Letter:* "The inositol hexaniacinate form of niacin has not been linked with the side effects associated with niacin supplementation. In a group of people being treated alternatively with niacin and inositol hexaniacinate for skin problems, niacin supplementation (50–100 mg per day) was associated with numerous side effects, including skin flushing, nausea, vomiting and agitation. In contrast, people taking inositol hexaniacinate experienced no complaints whatsoever, even at amounts two to five times higher than the previously used amounts of niacin."[8]

Dr. Jeffrey Baker, MD, an integrative family practitioner at the Immanuel Clinic in Springdale, AR, told me:

My first choice for reducing cholesterol is inositol hexaniacinate with a specific variety of antioxidants. I prescribe 600 mg twice daily. I believe the twice-daily approach is better than once-daily niacin therapies. I use inositol hexanicotinate a lot, and none of my patients have developed liver enzyme elevations.

In contrast, many mainstream doctors stick with prescription Niaspan and shy away from products not approved by the FDA because in the early 1980s, a popular, over-the-counter sustained-release niacin product was associated with liver toxicities. But that was not inositol hexaniacinate, which, despite widespread use, has not shown any of these problems. Indeed, according to another in-depth review in the *Alternative Medicine Review*, "No adverse effects have been reported from the use of inositol hexaniacinate in dosages as high as four grams daily."[15] Studies dating back 40 years have demonstrated the effectiveness and safety of inositol hexaniacinate for a variety of cardiovascular disorders.

The actual mechanism of action of inositol hexaniacinate is not clear. Originally it was thought that when the body slowly metabolizes a molecule of inositol hexaniacinate over twelve hours, it releases niacin (nicotinate acid) molecules. However, recent analyses suggest that little nicotinic acid is actually released in the blood of people taking inositol hexaniacinate. Because of this finding, some critics assert that inositol hexaniacinate should not be considered niacin. Nevertheless, whatever its exact mechanism of action, inositol hexaniacinate seems to have the same beneficial effects on elevated levels of cholesterol and other risk factors as standard niacin preparations.

Inositol hexaniacinate is usually started at 500 mg/day, then increased gradually to 1,000–2,000 mg/day. Inositol hexaniacinate should not be used by people with a history of liver disease. Liver enzyme levels should be checked when cholesterol levels are checked, especially if you are using doses above 2,000 mg/day. Inositol hexaniacinate is not FDA approved for treating lipid disorders or cardiovascular disease.

WHICH TYPE OF NIACIN SHOULD YOU USE?

Good doctors disagree about this. Cardiologist Stephen Sinatra, who knows the mainstream and alternative methods for reducing cholesterol about as well as anyone, prefers Niaspan, usually at doses of 750 to 1,500 mg/day. But among his recommendations he adds: "Since therapeutic levels of niacin can cause an unpleasant flushing sensation and headache, gradually increase your dosage over several weeks or use the flush-free form of niacin, inositol hexaniacinate."[16]

Alternative physician Dr. Whitaker prefers inositol hexanicotinate, usually at 500 mg three times a day, but up to 1,000 mg three times a day (with close medical monitoring). Most integrative medicine practitioners I know prefer inositol hexaniacinate, while many mainstream doctors have been taught that inositol hexanicotinate does not work. My experience is that it does.

My viewpoint is that unless you have acute cardiovascular disease, why not try inositol hexaniacinate first? It is far less expensive than prescription Niaspan, and inositol hexaniacinate appears to be freer of the vexing side effects of Niaspan or Endur-acin. If inositol hexaniacinate is not effective for you, you and your doctor can still consider Endur-acin or Niaspan. Whichever form of niacin is chosen, whether prescription or over the counter, I advise working closely with a healthcare practitioner. You will need to get blood tests anyway to know whether your cholesterol and/or other risk factors have been brought within target levels. Achieving your target levels is too important to undertake blindly. Niacin preparations can affect glucose, uric acid, and liver enzyme levels, so these should be checked too.

POLICOSANOL (EXTRACT OF SUGAR CANE)

Policosanol burst on the alternative medicine scene in early 2002. Its arrival was accompanied by an unusual amount of scientific evidence for a nutriceutical.

In a series of well-designed double-blind, placebo-controlled studies conducted in Cuba, where policosanol was developed, the substance lowered total cholesterol and LDL-C, while raising HDL-C:

- *American Heart Journal:* A review of 21 studies found that 10–20 mg of policosanol lowered total cholesterol 17 percent to 21 percent; LDL-C, 21 percent to 29 percent; and raised HDL-C 8 percent to 15 percent, on average, with few side effects. The authors concluded "Policosanol seems to be a very promising phytochemical alternative to classic lipid-lowering agents such as the statins."[17]

- *Current Therapeutics and Research:* In this double-blind, placebo-controlled study, 5 mg once daily of policosanol reduced LDL-C 17.7 percent on average.[18]

- *Current Therapeutics and Research:* In a double-blind, placebo-controlled study, 5 mg twice daily of policosanol reduced LDL-C 21.5 percent on average.[19]

- *Current Therapeutics and Research:* In a double-blind, placebo-controlled study, 5 mg twice daily of policosanol reduced LDL-C 21.2 percent, and 10 mg twice daily reduced LDL-C 30 percent on average.[20]

Policosanol has also been studied head to head against statins:

- *International Journal of Clinical Pharmacologic Research:* In this comparative double-blind trial, 10 mg of policosanol reduced LDL-C 19.3 percent on average; 10 mg of Pravachol reduced LDL-C 15.6 percent.[21]

- *Current Therapeutics and Research:* In a comparative, double-blind trial in elderly patients, 10 mg of policosanol reduced LDL-C 17.9 percent; 10 mg of Zocor reduced LDL-C 19.8 percent on average.[22]

- *Current Therapeutics and Research:* In a comparative,

double-blind trial in patients with coronary risk factors, 10 mg of policosanol reduced LDL-C 32.4 percent; 20 mg of Mevacor reduced LDL-C 27.6 percent on average.[23]

These and many other studies are impressive, yet it is important to remember that policosanol is relatively new. New chemicals—supplements as well as prescription drugs—should always be assessed carefully for their effectiveness. Moreover, "natural" does not automatically mean "safe." Because policosanol is relatively new to America, doctors in the U.S. have only limited experience with it. Jacqueline Campbell, MD, of Jamaica, has been using policosanol for many years: "In my practice I have used policosanol. We get it directly from Cuba. I have found 10 mg to be very effective in lowering total cholesterol levels."

The starting dose of policosanol is 5 or 10 mg/day, taken with dinner. A 20 mg dose is used for greater LDL-C reductions. Policosanol has no effect on triglycerides, and its effect on CRP is unknown. Policosanol is a mixture of alcohols (octacosanol, triacontanol, hexacosanol) isolated from purified sugar cane. Policosanol contains no sugar itself, so it can be used by diabetics. Policosanol appears to inhibit the production of cholesterol in the liver, but it does so differently than statins and does not seem to inhibit coenzyme A or deplete coenzyme Q_{10}. Policosanol also reduces LDL-C oxidation (oxidation makes LDL-C more harmful to arteries), and it reduces platelet aggregation by inhibiting thromboxane B_2 and the smooth muscle proliferation that may also play roles in the formation of atherosclerosis.[17]

Studies show that policosanol improves cardiac function, reduces angina symptoms, and increases endurance in people with severe atherosclerosis in the legs.[24]

So far, policosanol appears to be quite safe. In long-term studies, side effects were infrequent and minor (headache, dizziness, nervousness, insomnia, sedation, stomach pain, increased urination), but alternative doctors report few, if any, problems.[24] It remains to be seen, however, whether policosanol is as good as advertised. Already there are reports that Americans do not derive as much benefit as the Cuban studies indicate. Some doctors report mixed results, with some patients responding well, and other patients not responding. Other doctors say flatly that the policosanol available here does not work. Explanations for this include Americans' size or diets, or their more serious cholesterol problems. Another explanation involves manufacturing practices.

In America, most policosanol was originally derived from beets or beeswax instead of from sugar cane, which is the source of policosanol in Cuba. Because of the problems here, some American nutriceutical manufacturers are now producing policosanol from sugar cane with reportedly better results in patients. Nevertheless, Dr. Peter Jones of McGill University recently told a seminar audience that his group found no benefit in a carefully controlled study of high-quality sugar cane-derived policosanol.[25] Thus, the controversy continues.

Policosanol may be worth trying if its potential benefits fit your treatment goals, and if you can obtain the sugar cane-based product. The cost is low: about

$15–$30/month. Like red yeast rice, policosanol should be used with medical supervision. Policosanol is not FDA approved for reducing cholesterol or treating cardiovascular disease.

PLANT STEROLS (PHYTOSTEROLS)

Plant sterols are recommended by the American Heart Association and the National Cholesterol Education Program Expert Panel as adjunct therapy to reduce LDL.[26]
—AMERICAN JOURNAL OF MANAGED CARE

Sterols are essential components of the cell membranes of animals and plants. In humans, cholesterol is the main sterol. Plants manufacture other sterols. When people eat plant sterols or their derivatives (plant stanols), these substances impair the absorption of cholesterol from the intestine. Studies have shown that 1.5 to 2.5 grams/day of plant sterols reduces LDL-C by 10 percent on average (range: 6 percent to 14 percent).[27,28] Higher doses provide little extra benefit. These LDL-C reductions are comparable to those obtained with prescription drugs that block cholesterol absorption such as cholestyramine, Welchol, and Zetia, and plant sterols are less expensive and less side-effect prone. Like Zetia and Welchol, plant sterols can be used with statin drugs, which together can sometimes produce such good cholesterol reduction that the statin dosage can be reduced substantially.

According to Dr. Peter Jones, who is an expert on lipid metabolism, plant sterols are the most widely researched natural therapy for reducing cholesterol. Dr. Jones calls plant sterols "the best natural therapy for lowering cholesterol."[25] An article in the *Medical Journal of Australia* stated that "phytosterol-containing foods are valuable additions to other cholesterol-lowering treatments, including statins."[29] The *Journal of Nutrition* concurred: "It has been demonstrated that foods enriched with plant sterols and stanols are effective in various population groups, and in combination with cholesterol-lowering diets or drugs."[30] This is why both the National Institutes of Health and the U.S. Food and Drug Administration support the use of plant sterols for lowering cholesterol and reducing the risk of heart disease. An effective amount of plant sterols is 1.5 to 2.5 grams/day.

Plant sterols are present in small amounts in vegetable oils, seeds, nuts, some vegetables, and fruits. Margarines enriched with plant sterols are available today, but these should be avoided if they contain trans fats. You can buy supplements with plant sterols and stanols in health food stores. Plant sterols appear to cause few side effects in humans. There is some evidence that they may block the absorption of fat-soluble vitamins, especially carotene, which can be offset by an extra portion of an orange or yellow vegetable or fruit. The long-term effects of plant sterols are not known.

FIBER

There are two types of fiber: soluble and insoluble. Soluble fiber breaks down within the digestive tract and is absorbed into the body, while insoluble fiber passes through the intestines essentially unchanged. Soluble fiber can lower blood cholesterol and triglyceride levels. For example, oat bran can lower cholesterol 10 percent to 15 percent while reducing blood sugar and providing roughage for bowel health. Both types of fiber can reduce hypertension and blood glucose levels.[31] Both types of fiber have been shown to reduce the risk of heart disease, and insoluble fiber is associated with reduced risks of diverticulitis, and colon and breast cancer.

Dietary fiber comes from the thick cell walls of plants. Whole grains are good sources of insoluble fiber. Both types of fiber can be obtained from oats, barley, beans, vegetables, legumes, and whole fruit. Unfortunately, the typical Western diet is low in fiber content, providing about 10 grams of fiber per day. Our ancestors got 40 to 60 grams of fiber a day from their unprocessed foods. The FDA, the National Academy of Sciences, and the American Cancer Society recommend 25 to 35 grams of fiber per day.

Dr. Andrew Weil recommends dietary fiber among his cardiovascular health strategies: "Soluble fiber has a powerful cholesterol-lowering effect. The best sources of soluble fiber are beans and lentils, apple, citrus fruits, oats, barley, peas, carrots."[32] Packaged forms of soluble fiber include psyllium and pectin. The use of psyllium has been shown to allow statin patients to use lower statin doses. Chitosan, a new form of fiber derived from shellfish, has also produced some good initial results.

GUGGULIPID (GUGGUL, GUGUL)

Guggulipid is an extract of Gum guggul, a natural Ayurvedic medicine used in India for centuries. Guggulipid not only reduces cholesterol, but also acts as an antioxidant and reduces platelet aggregation. According to the People's Pharmacy, a column in the *Los Angeles Times,* guggulipid is approved in India for lowering cholesterol and preventing heart disease. Guggulipid's active ingredient is guggulsterone. The mechanism of action is not clear, but guggulipid appears to block LDL-C production or transport, and may block the absorption of cholesterol from the intestine. Another explanation is that guggulipid facilitates the production of bile acids, thereby enhancing the removal of cholesterol from the body. Guggulipid does not appear to deplete coenzyme Q_{10}.

Most studies of guggulipid have been conducted in India:

- *Cardiovascular Drugs and Therapeutics:* In this double-blind, placebo-controlled study of guggulsterone 50 mg twice daily in 31 patients, guggulipid reduced total cholesterol by 11.7 percent; LDL-C, 12.5 percent; triglycerides, 12 percent.[33]

- *Journal of the Association of Physicians of India:* In this twelve-week open trial involving 205 patients, guggulipid, 500 mg three times a day, reduced total cholesterol 23.6 percent and triglycerides 22.6 percent on average. Only one patient reported side effects (stomach pain). In a second double-blind phase, 125 patients taking guggulipid were compared with 108 patients taking the prescription drug clofibrate. Guggulipid reduced total cholesterol 11 percent and triglycerides 16.8 percent on average. Clofibrate reduced total cholesterol 10 percent and triglycerides 21.6 percent.[34]

Most striking about the latter study is the difference in cholesterol reduction—24 percent versus 11 percent—achieved in the study's two phases. Interestingly, doctors tell me the same thing. Some doctors report excellent results with guggulipid, while others don't. Dr. Baker told me, "I haven't seen impressive results. Other alternative methods work better." Yet, a review in the *American Family Physician* concluded that preliminary results with guggulipid are promising and toxicities appear to be few.[4] The operative word was "preliminary," because very few studies had been done. This changed in 2003 with the publication of the first major study in Western patients taking guggulipid.

In this double-blind study, 103 patients received 1,000 or 2,000 mg of guggulipid three times a day or placebo. The results: guggulipid actually raised LDL-C levels slightly and had no beneficial effect on total cholesterol, triglycerides, or HDL-C. Moreover, six people developed rashes with guggulipid compared to none with placebo.[35] When asked about the results, Dr. Philippe O. Szapary, who led the study, said, "The bottom line is, if you are trying to lower your [cholesterol], don't use guggulipid. There are plenty of proven safe and effective therapies on the market. We need to spend time and money investigating these products."[36] That is true, but no supplement manufacturer has the deep pockets of the drug companies, so studies on non-drug alternatives are sporadic.

This study made health-page headlines, and the articles were distinctly negative about guggulipid. Yet, a close reading of the published study revealed that high-dose guggulipid reduced median levels of CRP by 25 percent, which I confirmed in correspondence with Dr. Szapary (personal communication).[37] This is a significant and important finding, especially because CRP went up 30 percent in the placebo group. Low-dose guggulipid had no effect on CRP. Because more and more doctors believe that the inflammation reflected by CRP measurements is as important a risk factor as LDL-C levels, the impact of high-dose guggulipid on CRP may explain its long use in Ayurvedic medicine.

Where does this leave guggulipid as a treatment for atherosclerosis? On uncertain ground. Guggulipid may have an important role in reducing CRP, and in some patients, it may have beneficial effects on cholesterol levels. Because of the uncertainty, guggulipid should be used with medical monitoring of cholesterol and CRP levels.

The standard dose of guggulipid is 250 or 500 mg twice daily with meals; 500 mg three times a day is also used. Or, 25 mg of guggulsterone is used three times a day with meals. Side effects include nausea, gas, and bloating. Guggulipid is not FDA approved for reducing cholesterol or CRP, or for treating cardiovascular disease.

GARLIC

Garlic is said to reduce LDL-C and triglyceride levels, and to prevent the harmful oxidation of LDL-C. However, studies on garlic's cholesterol-lowering abilities are mixed. A 1994 review of garlic studies showed that garlic reduced total cholesterol by 12 percent.[38] However, in recent studies, garlic's effects have been less impressive. A study using two different doses of a garlic supplement showed no effect with the lower dose and a 6.1

percent reduction in total cholesterol with the higher dose.[39] A study of Kyolic garlic showed a modest 4 percent reduction in LDL-C; more impressive was its reduction of systolic blood pressure by 5.5 percent.[40]

A comprehensive review of garlic studies in the *Annals of Internal Medicine* found that garlic reduced cholesterol levels by 7 percent on average. The authors concluded: "The available data suggest that garlic is superior to placebo in reducing total cholesterol levels. However, the size of the effect is modest." They concluded that using garlic to reduce cholesterol levels was "questionable."[41] An article in the *American Family Physician* went further:

> Despite the many early promising studies and meta-analyses evaluating garlic's effect as a lipid-lowering agent, more recent, rigorous studies have failed to substantiate these benefits. There is no current role for garlic as an antihyperlipidemic agent.[4]

Garlic's effects on cholesterol levels and blood pressure may be modest on average, but some people attest to getting good results. Dr. Whitaker states, "Garlic promotes an optimum ratio of LDL-to-HDL cholesterol and promotes elastic artery walls ."[42] He recommends garlic in combinations with guggulipid, flax, niacin, and B vitamins. Dr. Weil recommends fresh garlic: "Garlic has been shown to lower both cholesterol levels and blood pressure—and it tastes wonderful, too. Use one or two lightly cooked cloves a day."[32]

The usual dosage of garlic is 400–600 mg per day, although this may differ with different formulations. Garlic's safety is established, and its cost is low. Even with modest results, garlic can serve as an adjunct to other methods of reducing cholesterol, allowing you to use lower doses of cholesterol-lowering drugs or other supplements. In addition, garlic is believed to have some antibacterial properties, and many alternative doctors include garlic in their regimens for reducing blood pressure.

Garlic is not FDA approved for reducing cholesterol or treating cardiovascular disease. Garlic can cause mild inhibition of platelets, which can be compounded if you are also using ginkgo biloba or fish oils. Because of its platelet-inhibition properties, garlic should be discontinued at least one week before surgery.

SOY

The FDA has approved this health claim:

> 25 grams of soy protein a day, as part of a diet low in saturated fat and cholesterol, may reduce the risk of heart disease.[43]

Indeed, studies dating back as far as 1941 have demonstrated soy's beneficial effects on cholesterol levels. Studies show that soy protein reduces total cholesterol about 9 percent; LDL-C, 13 percent; and triglycerides, 10 percent, on average.[4,44,45] But soy's effect on these factors is variable: some people obtain substantial cholesterol reductions, others don't. New evidence suggests that soy may also favorably influence the size of LDL-C particles.[46]

Getting 25 grams of soy protein daily is not easy. Two ounces of tofu contains 8.5 grams of soy protein, and there are just so many soy burgers and soy hot dogs you can eat. Soy milk, soy flour, soy puddings, and supplements are other ways of getting soy.

However, some experts have expressed concern about using soy in large quantities. Dr. Sherry Rogers, a leading voice in alternative medicine, does not recommend soy because of its estrogenic effects. Drs. Daniel Sheehan and Daniel Doerge, FDA experts on soy, argued against approving the soy health statement because of soy's effects on estrogen-sensitive tissues and the thyroid.[47] Joseph Mercola, MD, who produces one of the most popular health websites in the world (www.mercola.com), is not fond of soy: "Soy is not the health food that it's made out to be. I regularly see women who have thyroid problems as a result of consuming soy."[48]

Other doctors strongly disagree and recommend moderate amounts of soy and believe it can play a role in heart health and longevity. Dr. Whitaker states:

> Soybeans are an excellent source of high-quality protein, fiber, sterols, and specialized phytonutrients known as isoflavones, powerful antioxidants that protect the arteries, lower cholesterol, discourage LDL-C oxidation, and help prevent the formation of potentially dangerous blood clots.

Whitaker acknowledges that some doctors disagree, but adds, "I've looked at this issue from every angle, and I remain convinced that the good outweighs the bad."[49] He recommends that people eat soy several times a week.

An analysis in *Consumer Reports* concluded:

> A large body of evidence shows that soy can be good for most people. Soy protein, which can help lower

cholesterol and reduce the risk of heart attack, contains the nine essential amino acids found in animal protein, but it is much lower in saturated fat and has no cholesterol.

Noting the FDA's approval of soy and that 25 mg/day of soy protein can lower total cholesterol by 5 percent to 10 percent, the magazine added "such reductions should produce a 10% to 30% drop in heart attack risk."[50]

It would be comforting if this was the last word, but around the same time, the *Los Angeles Times* stated "soy has been losing luster for years."[51] The emerging research on soy has not upheld the FDA's health claim, according to Alice Lichtenstein, a professor of nutrition science at Tufts University. Soy, she stated, has "very little effect" on lowering LDL-C.[51] Yet, Dr. Stephen Pratt, in his best-seller *Superfoods*, lists soy as one of the top fourteen foods you can eat. Dr. Pratt specifically mentions soy's potential to reduce cholesterol.[52]

Clearly, the final chapter on soy remains to be written. In the meantime, you can try soy products and see whether they help reduce your total cholesterol and LDL-C levels. It may be that soy is helpful for some, but not others. If you get a 5-percent to 10-percent reduction from soy, and you combine this with other nutritional and other lifestyle efforts, you will be doing a lot to maintain cardiovascular health.

PANTETHINE

Pantethine is a natural substance formed during the body's metabolism of pantothenic acid (vitamin B_5). A series of studies have shown that pantethine can produce moderate reductions in levels of total cholesterol, LDL-C, and triglycerides.[53–55] Some patients also obtained increases in HDL-C. The mechanism by which pantethine works is unclear, but may be due to inhibition of cholesterol production in the liver. Pantethine is also said to reduce platelet clumping by inhibiting the production of the pro-inflammatory substance thromboxane A2. The usual dosage of pantethine is 300 mg three times daily. At higher dosages, pantethine has been used for treating the burning pain of peripheral neuropathies. Studies have reported no serious side effects.

TOCOTRIENOLS

Tocotrienols are natural constituents of palm and rice bran oils. Although similar in structure to vitamin E (tocopherols), tocotrienols possess unique antioxidant qualities. Tocotrienols have been reported to reduce cholesterol and LDL-C by inhibiting the same liver enzyme (HMG-Co-A reductase) involved in cholesterol synthesis that is inhibited by statin drugs. However, clinical studies of tocotrienols have produced mixed results. One group has published several studies demonstrating significant cholesterol reduction with tocotrienols,[56,57] but studies by other researchers have shown no benefit on cholesterol or LDL-C levels.[58–60] I asked ten integrative physicians if they recommend tocotrienols for cholesterol reduction. None use tocotrienols for this purpose, but because of their potent antioxidant effects, several practitioners recommend a combination of alpha and gamma vitamin E plus tocotrienols in dosages of 100 to 400 IU per day.

BUYING SUPPLEMENTS THAT WORK

The major drawback to non-drug alternatives is that the manufacturing is not regulated, and studies have shown that some supplement products do not contain the amounts claimed on their labels. For example, in a study published in the *Archives of Internal Medicine*, 28 of 59 preparations (47 percent) of the herb echinacea did not contain the amounts listed on the labels, and six preparations (10 percent) contained no echinacea at all. Products that claimed to be standardized were no more reliable than others.[61]

Some years ago, Dr. Sinatra encountered similar variability when he first began using coenzyme Q_{10} with patients. Responses were so variable, Dr. Sinatra sent samples of his patients' pills for laboratory assay. Many pills contained far less than the 30 mg claimed on the packages. One pill contained just 1 mg of CoQ_{10}.[62]

Manufacturing practices are improving in the nutriceutical industry, and many companies now produce their products according to pharmaceutical quality guidelines, and have their products assessed by independent laboratories. Still, product quality can vary from company to company, so I advise people to buy supplements made by reputable companies with long track records. Your alternative doctor can also recommend products with which he or she has obtained good results. Also, by monitoring your cholesterol or CRP levels, it should be apparent whether the supplement is working. It may be cheaper to buy bargain supplements, but getting effective treatment is far more important than saving a few pennies a day. Whether online or in a health food store, stick with products from well-known, reputable companies.

As this chapter demonstrates, there are many natural therapies that can be used with or instead of statin medications. Research studies and clinical experience with patients demonstrate that the most reliable for reducing cholesterol are red yeast rice (which should not be used with statins), niacin or inositol hexaniacinate, plant sterols, and fiber. Possibly effective for reducing cholesterol are guggulipid and pantethine. The evidence for policosanol and tocotrienols is mixed, so their effectiveness remains questionable and results may vary from person to person. Other natural therapies that are sometimes mentioned as being helpful for lowering cholesterol include artichoke extract, cinnamon, citrulline, citrus bioflavenoids, phosphatidylcholine (the main constituent of lecithin), and raw almonds. Although all of these therapies can be obtained without a prescription, I advise people to work with a knowledgeable healthcare provider in deciding among the many choices and doses of these natural therapies, and in monitoring their effects on cholesterol levels, CRP, and other risk factors.

The Four Essential Nutrients for Cardiovascular Health

More than half of the 1.1 million heart attacks that are suffered in the U.S. annually occur in people who do not have elevated cholesterol. Clearly, there is a lot more to maintaining heart health than simply taking a cholesterol-lowering pill. Even if you take a statin drug, it does not provide full protection. Statins reduce the risk of heart attacks by 30 percent, which means that 70 percent of the risk still exists. Statins may lower cholesterol and LDL-C, but the drugs do not restore health to an unhealthy vascular system or improve deficiencies of key nutrients. Therefore, whether you take a cholesterol-lowering agent or not, it is important to consider other methods that can help you maintain the optimal functioning of your heart and blood vessels.

People usually think of the substances discussed in this chapter—omega-3 oils, coenzyme Q_{10}, folic acid, and magnesium—as supplements, but they aren't. They are nutrients, requisite parts of our physiology, needed by human cells and structures just like amino acids or vitamin C, and necessary for proper body functioning. Yet many people are severely deficient in omega-3 oils and magnesium, and coenzyme Q_{10} and folic acid are particularly important for cardiovascular health, yet they are routinely ignored in mainstream medicine today.

OMEGA-3 FATTY ACIDS (FISH OILS, ESSENTIAL FATTY ACIDS)

Failure to eat enough essential fatty acids is a cause of hardening of the arteries, abnormal clot formation, coronary heart disease, high cholesterol, and high blood pressure.[1]
—EDWARD SIEGEL, MD, PHD

Omega-3 fatty acids (EPA and DHA) may be as important as any of the pharmaceuticals and nutriceuticals discussed in this book. The human body cannot make all of the kinds of fats it requires. Some are essential: they must be obtained from foods. These essential oils are linolenic and linoleic, which provide omega-3 and omega-6 fatty acids, respectively. Omega-3 and omega-6 fatty acids serve many vital functions in the body, and one of their foremost functions is to maintain cardiovascular health. Together, omega-3 and omega-6 fatty acids reduce LDL-C and raise HDL-C. Higher doses of omega-3 oils also reduce triglyceride levels. But it is not that simple, because in Western countries today, most people get too many omega-6 oils from corn, soy, safflower, sunflower, peanut, and cottonseed oils that are used so widely in packaged foods, salad dressings, and fast foods. Worse, very few people get enough omega-3 fatty oils, which are plentiful only in fatty fish (sardines, ocean salmon, swordfish, and tuna that isn't nonfat) and flax seeds, and getting enough omega-3 oils is fundamental to maintaining cardiovascular health.

The importance of omega-3 oils did not become well known until the late 1990s, and a lot of people still have not gotten the word. Scientists did not know about omega-3 oils either until the late 1970s, when studies showed that Eskimos, despite fat-laden diets, had substantially fewer heart attacks than people in Western societies. These findings defied the accepted wisdom that excess fat in the diet causes atherosclerosis and heart disease. The observation that the fat from fish might be beneficial launched a new area of research, as described in the *Mayo Clinic Proceedings:*

> These observations generated more than 4,500 studies to explore this and other effects of omega-3 fatty acids on human metabolism and health. From epidemiology to cell culture and animal studies to randomized controlled trials, the cardioprotective effects of omega-3 fatty acids are becoming recognized.[2]

Such recognition has come slowly. It was not until a large, placebo-controlled Italian study, known as the GISSI study, was published in *Lancet* in 1999 that mainstream medicine began to take serious notice. In this study, more than 11,000 people with recent heart attacks were given 1 gram/day of omega-3 oils or placebo for three and a half years. Over just 3.5 years, the omega-3 group had significantly fewer heart attacks and strokes, cardiac death was reduced 45 percent, and death from all causes was reduced 20 percent.[3] Today, it is widely accepted that omega-3 fatty acids reduce heart attacks, strokes, and deaths from heart disease, as well as the overall incidence of death from all causes.

We also know that omega-3 oils are a critical factor

Evidence-Based Information on the Benefits of Omega-3 Fatty Acids

Here is a small sample of the many articles in the medical literature about the benefits of omega-3 fatty acids.

- *European Heart Journal:* "Sudden cardiac death is very common ...and accounts for about 50% of cardiovascular mortality in developed countries. . . . Clinical and epidemiological studies, and randomized trials, clearly demonstrated that omega-3 polyunsaturated fatty acids reduce the risk of sudden cardiac death. Their clinical use is now encouraged."[4]

- *New England Journal of Medicine:* "The omega-3 fatty acids found in fish are strongly associated with a reduced risk of sudden death among men without evidence of prior cardiovascular disease." Compared to men with the lowest levels of omega-3 fatty acids, the men in this study with the highest levels of omega-3s "had an 81 percent lower risk of sudden death."[5]

- *JAMA:* "Among women, higher consumption of fish and omega-3 fatty acids is associated with a lower risk of

in keeping blood vessels functioning properly and in preventing cardiac arrhythmias when heart attacks occur. For many people, the first symptom of heart disease is a heart attack. Each year, 250,000 people die from sudden cardiac death, usually from heart attacks that are not in themselves lethal, but which trigger arrhythmias that are. Multiple studies have now proven that omega-3 oils reduce the risk of sudden cardiac death by an astounding 40 percent to 80 percent (see the insert on coronary heart disease, particularly coronary heart disease deaths. . . . In our study, omega-3 fatty acid intake and fish consumption were associated with a significantly lower risk of coronary heart disease."[6]

• *Circulation:* "A growing consensus for a direct relationship between increased intake of omega-3 fatty acids either from dietary sources or as a pharmacological supplementation and decreasing risk of coronary heart disease has become apparent over the years." This study: "Patients allocated to omega-3 fatty acids treatment had a significantly lower mortality even after only 3 months of treatment."[7]

• *Public Health and Nutrition:* "For decades it has been postulated that the main environmental factor for coronary heart disease was the intake of saturated fatty acids. Nevertheless, confirmation of the role of saturated fatty acids in coronary heart disease through intervention trials has been disappointing. It was only when the diet was enriched with omega-3 fatty acids that coronary heart disease was significantly prevented, especially cardiac death."[8]

pages 64–65).[4–9] "The higher your blood level of omega-3, the lower your risk" of sudden cardiac death, says Dr. Christine M. Albert, the chief of cardiology at Massachusetts General Hospital and the lead author of a major study on this issue.[5]

Despite these proven benefits, mainstream doctors often fail to suggest omega-3 oils to patients. And despite headlines in the mainstream media about studies proving the benefits of omega-3 oils, this issue is not mentioned when famous people die suddenly from heart attacks. In the sports world in 2002 and 2003, lethal heart attacks struck Johnny Unitas (football), 32-year-old Darryl Kile (baseball), and Dave DeBusschere (basketball)—all former all-stars. Yet, in the stories about these legends' deaths, not a question was asked about their diets or their intakes of fish or omega-3 oils. Not a word was written that these deaths might have been preventable. So what I call the Unitas-Kile-DeBusschere Syndrome—sudden cardiac death—continues to go unrecognized and uncorrected in our society. This is unfortunate, because most Westerners are deficient in omega-3 oils, and eating fatty fish once weekly or taking two to three fish oil capsules a day is not only recommended by the Expert U.S. Panel and the British Nutrition Foundation, but also easy and inexpensive.

Because they are essential nutrients, omega-3 oils have many other benefits. Omega-3 oils improve the functioning of the endothelium lining the insides of arteries. Omega-3 oils have anti-inflammatory effects that may be helpful in reducing C-reactive protein levels and preventing artery damage and atherosclerosis. Studies have shown that men with high levels of arterial inflammation are far more likely to have heart attacks and strokes than men with low levels of inflammation.[10,11] Omega-3 oils are the body's natural anti-inflammatory substances. Omega-3 oils also inhibit platelet clumping and the clotting that contributes to coronary disease and strokes. These properties are reasons why the American Heart Association recommends at least two servings of fish a week.[12]

Due to their anti-inflammatory effect, high doses of

omega-3 oils have proven beneficial in studies of autoimmune disorders such as rheumatoid arthritis and Crohn's disease, so omega-3s should also help reduce CRP. Yet studies of omega-3 oils for CRP have been equivocal, probably because the doses studied were inadequate. Authorities recommend 2–3 grams/day of fish oil to reduce cardiac arrhythmias, but inflammatory disorders like rheumatoid arthritis or lupus require 6–12 grams/day. These higher doses may also be necessary for reducing elevated CRP. The studies on omega-3 oils for CRP may also have been too brief. Correcting deficiencies of omega-3 oils takes time. Restoring the balance of essential oils in all of your 50 trillion cells cannot be done overnight. This usually takes four to six months, and also requires a reduction in pro-inflammatory omega-6 oils.

Omega-3 oils are something on which mainstream and alternative doctors agree. Dr. Andrew Weil says, "The omega-3 fatty acids in fish and fish oil supplements have been shown to be an effective preventive strategy against heart disease. They can lower triglycerides levels, increase HDL-C, help minimize inflammation and blood clotting, and keep blood vessels healthy."[13] Cardiologist Stephen Sinatra, MD, adds, "The EPA contained in fish oil is a terrific anti-inflammatory agent. And the DHA in fish oil has been shown to help minimize asthma and arthritis, along with inflammation caused by cancer."[14]

Indeed, omega-3 oils also may help prevent cancer of the breast, colon, and prostate. Omega-3 oils improve glucose metabolism, reduce insulin reactivity, and reduce blood pressure. Omega-3 oils reduce triglyceride levels, but have variable effects on LDL-C. But when taken with a small amount of gamma-linoleic acid (GLA), an omega-6 fatty acid, LDL-C levels are reduced.

How can you get more omega-3 oils? Some experts recommend eating fatty fish once or twice a week to obtain the heart benefits, but others discourage this because of toxins that accumulate in the fat of these fish. The FDA already warns pregnant women against eating too much fish because of the effects of mercury on developing children, and that was before 2003, when the FDA lowered its safety standard for mercury in humans to one-quarter its previous amount. High levels of mercury have also been associated with infertility.[15] Dr. Joseph Mercola recommends avoiding most fish:

> Some fish have less mercury than others, but nearly all fish are contaminated with mercury. I have done thousands of hair mineral analyses on patients. . . [and] patients who don't eat any fish are the only ones who have immeasurable levels of mercury in their hair. Anyone eating fish has mercury in their system, and it is nearly always in direct proportion to the frequency of their fish consumption.

Exceptions: sardines and anchovies have little mercury, probably because they have not been in the ocean long enough to accumulate a lot in their tissues.[16] Other experts disagree with Dr. Mercola's perspective and contend that a moderate intake of fish is safe and beneficial.

Do the fish you eat actually contain omega-3 oils? Much of the salmon offered at markets today is farmed. These fish receive feeds that are not like the natural plankton eaten by wild fish and do not stimulate the production of as much omega-3 oils. Moreover, a recent report showed higher levels of toxins in farmed fish. So if you want to eat fish in order to obtain omega-3 oils, choose wild ocean fish.

Early man had no difficulty getting enough omega-3 oils. His diet relied on free ranging animals, which manufactured omega-3 oils naturally from the grasses they ate. Modern man gets meat from animals raised on grains, which are not their natural foods and do not allow their bodies to produce much omega-3 oil. This is why alternative doctors like Dr. Mercola now recommend range-raised beef, whose main feed is grass.

The easiest and most reliable way of getting enough omega-3 oils is from fish oil capsules. Quality is the key here, and high-quality capsules have had the omega-3 oils cleaned and detoxified of metals, pesticides, and other toxins. Then the oils are combined with a little vitamin E to maintain freshness. High-quality fish oil capsules should have no odor or fishy taste. A gram of fish oil usually provides 300 mg of omega-3 oils (EPA and DHA). Some companies are making more potent capsules containing 500 mg of omega-3 oils, meaning fewer capsules and fewer calories. Others are marketing potent capsules containing only DHA, but I prefer capsules with a balance of EPA and DHA.

In order to maximize the anti-inflammatory effects of omega-3 oils, you may have to reduce your intake of pro-inflammatory omega-6 oils. The idea of limiting omega-6 oils is controversial. Some experts disagree with limiting omega-6 oils, but Dr. Artemis Simopoulos, who for decades has been the foremost researcher and educator about omega-3 oils, recommends limiting omega-6s. Studies of autoimmune diseases also suggest that limiting omega-6 oils while increasing omega-3s is necessary for reducing inflammation.

The fact is most people are already saturated with omega-6 oils. Healthy diets should provide a ratio of omega-6:omega-3 oils of 2:1 or 1:1, but Western diets are so imbalanced toward omega-6 oils, the ratio is closer to 17:1. People are supposed to get about 1 gram of omega-3 oils daily, but the average intake is about 0.1–0.2 grams/day. This dietary imbalance of too much pro-inflammatory omega-6 and too little anti-inflammatory omega-3 may explain why inflammatory diseases and inflammation of the arteries are so widespread today. To correct the balance, you need an omega-6:omega-3 intake that approaches 1:1.

Which oils can you use? Olive oil. Olive oil. Olive oil. Scores of studies of people eating Mediterranean diets rich in olive oil demonstrate much lower incidences of cardiovascular disease and much greater longevity. Olive oil contains many healthful constituents and is loaded with antioxidants. When olive oil cannot be used, I prefer canola oil, which does contain some omega-6 fatty acids but also contains omega-3s. Dr. Mercola recommends coconut oil for cooking because, despite its high saturated fat content, it does not break down when subjected to intense heat.

Do omega-3 oils have a downside? Large amounts of fish oils are said to increase bleeding tendencies, although reports of this are few, and none of the mainstream or alternative doctors I know who use fish oils have seen any problems. Nevertheless, fish oils should be used carefully with aspirin and are contraindicated with blood thinners. In fact, some people take fish oils instead of aspirin to prevent heart disease. While doctors strongly recommend daily low-dose aspirin for people with heart disease, aspirin is not recommended for others. Many people use aspirin anyway, but aspirin has its own risks such as gastric bleeding or increased bleeding from trauma such as automobile accidents. Fish oils may offer a safer alternative. High doses of omega-3 oils should be taken with a doctor's supervision. If you are taking high doses of fish oil supplements, you should have your doctor check your cellular levels of omega-3 and omega-6 fatty acids with your annual laboratory tests. Fish oil supplements are not FDA approved for reducing cholesterol or treating cardiovascular disease.

COENZYME Q_{10}

Coenzyme Q_{10} (CoQ_{10}) is a powerful antioxidant that is found in every cell in the body. Coenzyme Q_{10} facilitates energy production in the mitochondria of cells, inhibits the oxidation of LDL-C, and has shown benefit in coronary disease, arrhythmias, congestive heart failure, and hypertension. Our cells make CoQ_{10}, but the ability to do so begins to fade after age forty. In healthy hearts, tissue levels of CoQ_{10} are much higher than in any other organ in the body. Because of the heart's high energy requirements, a deficiency in CoQ_{10} affects the heart more than any other organ and can contribute to development of congestive heart failure. Coenzyme Q_{10}'s benefits have been demonstrated in studies.

"Coenzyme Q_{10}—CoQ_{10}—the nutrient I can't imagine practicing medicine without," states Dr. Sinatra. "CoQ_{10} supports healthy HDL and prevents the excess oxidation of LDL." Dr. Sinatra recommends 45 to 90 mg of softgel CoQ_{10} daily, but much higher doses for people with congestive heart failure. He also recommends 30 to 90 mg/day of CoQ_{10} for women over 30, because women are more vulnerable than men to CoQ_{10} deficiency.[11]

Dr. Julian Whitaker concurs: "Every patient I treat who has heart disease is immediately placed on CoQ_{10}. CoQ_{10} deficiencies and heart failure go hand in hand, and patients with the lowest levels generally have the most severe disease."[17] Dr. Whitaker recounts cases in which CoQ_{10} produced remarkable improvement in people with severe, end-stage congestive heart failure. Dr. Whitaker has petitioned the FDA to require a warning in statin package inserts about the importance of taking coenzyme Q_{10} with statins.

Coenzyme Q_{10} is another extensively studied nutrient that mainstream doctors are just now learning about, but alternative doctors have been recommending for years. Many alternative doctors believe that the muscle pain and fatigue accompanying statin therapy is caused by statins' blocking of the body's production of CoQ_{10}, and they attest that CoQ_{10} reduces or eliminates these side effects. In fact, some alternative doctors prescribe statins, but when they do, they also recommend CoQ_{10}.

CoQ_{10} is not FDA approved for reducing cholesterol or treating cardiovascular disease.

FOLIC ACID

You can't say, 'Well, I'll take folic acid and eat whatever I want.' But I do recommend folic acid for all of my patients.[18]
—CRAIG SCOTT, MD

In the rush to embrace C-reactive protein as the explanation for why 50 percent of heart attacks occur in people with normal cholesterol levels, folic acid should not be forgotten. Folic acid does not reduce cholesterol, but it does reduce homocysteine, which, at elevated levels, is directly linked to coronary artery disease. Elevated homocysteine is also linked to an increased incidence of congestive heart failure.[19] The large National Health and Nutrition Examination Survey (NHANES I) found that low folic acid intakes were associated with higher rates of strokes and other cardiovascular disorders.[20]

Yet, doctors have long overlooked and underutilized folic acid for reducing people's cardiovascular risk. Elevated homocysteine levels have also been linked to impaired cognitive functioning and Parkinson's and Alzheimer's diseases in the elderly, pregnancy complications, birth defects, increased death rates in diabetics, and possibly cancer. As mentioned in Chapter 2, elevated homocysteine levels develop in people who are unable to fully metabolize the amino acid methionine, which is abundant in meat. Reducing the intake of animal protein can lower homocysteine levels. Folic acid, with B_{12} and low doses of B_6, is effective in facilitating the metabolism of methionine, thereby reducing homocysteine levels.

How much folic acid do you need? The U.S. Rec-

ommended Daily Allowance is 400 micrograms/day
(0.4 milligrams/day). However, for people with atherosclerosis, a study in the *American Journal of Hypertension*
found that 2.5 mg/day of folic acid, 0.25 mg B_{12}, plus 25
mg of B_6 reversed artery clogging.[21] Another study
found that older people need at least 1 mg/day of folic
acid for its cardiovascular benefits.[22] Some people may
need much larger doses. "About 30% of my patients with
elevated homocysteine don't use folic acid very effi-
ciently," states Dr. Neil Hirschenbein of La Jolla, CA.
"Some people need 10 or even 20 mg of folic acid a
day."[23]

Some people cannot metabolize folic acid to its
active form in their cells. If this is the case, you can
purchase the active form, L-5-MTHF (L-5-methyl tetra-
hydrofolate), from some supplement companies. Trimethylglycine (TMG) can also be used to reduce
homocysteine levels.

Although most doctors know that elevated homocysteine can damage blood vessels and cause narrow-
ing of arteries, relatively few doctors order homocysteine
levels for their patients. Ask your doctor about including a homocysteine level in your next blood study. Normal homocysteine levels are usually defined as up to 20
micromoles per liter (μmol/L) of plasma, but some
experts believe that a level above 9 is too high.[21] "Our
own laboratory still defines normal as below 20 micromoles," Dr. Mimi Guarneri, cardiologist and medical
director of the Scripps Clinic Center for Integrative
Medicine, stated at a recent conference. "But I believe
normal homocysteine levels are less than 9."

Some alternative doctors advise levels a bit lower: 7

or below. Hopefully, mainstream medicine and mainstream laboratories will get the word soon, because new studies suggest that for each 5 µmol/L elevation in homocysteine levels, cardiovascular risk increases by 60 percent in men and 80 percent in women.[24]

MAGNESIUM

Magnesium does not lower cholesterol or CRP, but it is so important for cardiac and vascular health, it must be mentioned. The medical literature is filled with hundreds upon hundreds of studies of magnesium's beneficial effects:

- *U.S. National Institutes of Health:* "Magnesium deficiency can cause metabolic changes that may contribute to heart attacks and strokes. Population surveys have associated higher blood levels of magnesium with lower risk of coronary heart disease . . . and of stroke."[25]

- *Medicinski Pregled* [*Medical Review (Croatia)*]: "It has been accepted by authors all over the world that the role of magnesium is of great importance in the prevention and treatment of cardiac patients."[26]

- *USA Weekend:* "Minus magnesium, hearts beat irregularly; arteries stiffen, constrict and clog; blood pressure rises; blood tends to clot; muscles spasm; insulin grows weaker and blood sugar jumps; bones lose strength; and pain signals intensify."[27]

- *African Journal of Medicine and Medical Science:* "Congestive heart failure is associated with electrolyte imbalance including magnesium deficit, which may increase myocardial electrical instability, risk of arrhythmias, and sudden death."[28]

There is an astonishing amount of scientific articles on magnesium. Magnesium's importance for general and cardiovascular health is indisputable. "Magnesium has a well-deserved reputation as the number 1 cardiovascular disease prevention mineral," states Jonathan Wright, MD, an early pioneer of the alternative medicine movement.[29] Cardiologist Sinatra adds, "Magnesium, the unsung hero of heart health, can be life-saving, especially for those who have suffered a heart attack or are at high risk; are prone to ventricular arrhythmias; are planning open-heart surgery; have congestive heart failure or cardiomyopathy; have high blood pressure; or are on long-term diuretics."[30] As many as 75 percent of people in Western societies are magnesium deficient, yet most mainstream doctors do not know about it, and standard magnesium tests are not accurate enough to show even major deficiencies. Most people do not get anywhere near the RDA of 320–400 mg of magnesium in their diets, and some experts believe that the RDA is too low. Alternative doctors often recommend 500–1,000 mg/day.

The best known magnesium supplements are inexpensive, inorganic salts such as magnesium oxide that are poorly absorbed, causing gas or diarrhea. However, getting enough magnesium is essential for treating many cardiovascular conditions including hypertension, Raynaud's phenomena, and migraines. In fact, although magnesium is rarely used by mainstream doctors for treating office patients, it is frequently used in urgent care centers because of its proven ability to relax blood vessels and to reduce excitability of heart and brain cells. Intravenous magnesium is used in cardiac care units for cardiac arrhythmias and on obstetrical floors for eclampsia, which causes acute hypertension and seizures in pregnant women.

Magnesium was the key to my overcoming a very rare, severe vascular disease known as erythromelalgia. After trying scores of drugs, medical procedures, and alternative methods that did not work, I finally got improvement with prescription calcium channel blockers. But even at modest doses, I could not handle their side effects and found, to my own edification, that magnesium worked better with no side effects. I also learned that magnesium is needed to balance calcium in blood vessels and muscles, thereby reducing muscle tension and nerve excitability. After having been disabled for years, magnesium gradually got me into remission that has lasted several years. As the Chairman of the Medical Advisory Committee of The Erythromelalgia Association, I have recommended magnesium to scores of people and have learned that magnesium helps some but not others. This is not surprising because of the great variability in response seen with most therapies for vascular diseases such as hypertension and migraines. The fact that magnesium helps about 50 percent—people who had not responded to dozens of other treatments—is pretty good, better and safer and far less expensive than many highly touted drugs.

I want to underscore the importance of magnesium in helping people prevent hypertension, which is the single greatest contributor to cardiovascular disease. How serious is this wear and tear cause by hypertension? *Conn's Current Therapy*, a leading medical reference, described it this way:

> A 35-year-old man with an arterial pressure of 130/90 will die 4 years earlier than another 35-year-old man with the same medical background but with normal pressure. If his pressure is 140/90, he will die 9 years earlier, and if it's 150/100, he will die 17 years earlier.[31]

Although this book focuses on maintaining cardiovascular health by reducing cholesterol, CRP, homocysteine, and other atherosclerosis-causing factors, hypertension is a more serious and more certain risk factor for vascular damage, heart attacks, and strokes than any of them. If you have hypertension and high cholesterol or high CRP and must treat one first, treat the hypertension. Magnesium is not a panacea, but like potassium, magnesium should be a first-line therapy for most cases of hypertension. It is especially important for people taking diuretics, which wash out magnesium. Magnesium may also be helpful in reducing the risk of cardiac arrhythmias and sudden cardiac death.

If you have mild-to-moderate hypertension, as 48 million Americans do, and you want to avoid medications, you may be able to do so with a heart-healthy diet, moderate weight loss (if needed), moderate exercise, adequate intake of potassium (which is plentiful in vegetables), moderate salt restriction, and supplementation with magnesium. Even if you do require medication, these steps will allow you to use lower doses and fewer drugs.

Because it is difficult to get enough magnesium even when you eat the right foods (beans, seafood, apricots, bananas, spinach, broccoli, sweet potatoes, seaweed, seeds), I recommend supplementation for most people. Start with 100 mg of magnesium twice daily with meals, then increase gradually. People who get diarrhea with standard magnesium oxide or other magnesium salts usually do fine with magnesium chelate. Absorption is best when magnesium is in solution (over-the-counter magnesium chloride solution), which makes it highly absorbable. Calcium-magnesium combinations are fine for healthy people, but for medical uses such as hypertension or migraines, magnesium may be more effective when taken alone than in multivitamins or in combination with other minerals.

Magnesium doses above the RDA should be taken with medical supervision. Seniors and people with kidney disease or who are taking medications for cardiovascular or neurological disorders should get medical supervision even for RDA doses.

Even for people who require a statin medication, there is a lot more to maintaining cardiovascular health than taking a prescription drug. The body is an intricate, amazing balance of natural substances, and your health depends on providing your body with the essential nutrients it needs. Supplements are one way to provide vital nutrients. Foods are another, and selecting the best heart-healthy diet for you is the subject of the next chapter.

WHICH HEART-HEALTHY DIET IS RIGHT FOR YOU? YOUR INDIVIDUALIZED, OPTIMUM DIET

> *In a rational healthcare system, we would begin with nutrition, then natural therapies, and then drugs only when necessary. Today, it is usually just the opposite. Drugs have a role, absolutely, but they are frequently used first even when nutrition or natural remedies may be the answer.*
> —JAY S. COHEN, MD, 2003

A large number of people diagnosed medically with high cholesterol, "hypercholesterolemia," do not have medical disorders at all. They have nutritional imbalances. As a society, it is irrational for us to be elevating our LDL-C levels and triglyceride levels, while lowering HDL-C levels, with bad nutrition, then defining these abnormal measurements as medical disorders and taking powerful cholesterol-lowering drugs that have serious risks and cost billions, while convincing ourselves that doing so is perfectly reasonable.

The preeminent role of good nutrition in reducing cardiovascular risk is not an alternative idea—it is emphasized in standard textbooks and drug references. Even package inserts and PDR descriptions of statin drugs acknowledge that diet comes first. For example, the dosage guidelines for Lipitor begin with: "The patient should be placed on a standard cholesterol-lowering diet before receiving Lipitor and should continue on this diet during treatment with Lipitor."[1] The American Hospital Formulary Service emphasizes the secondary role of statins to diet: "Statins are used as *adjuncts to dietary therapy* to reduce the risk of a first major acute coronary event."[2] (Emphasis added.) Indeed, studies have shown that a good diet can reduce cholesterol levels as much as a moderate-dose statin drug.

For example, a recent study in *JAMA* showed that diet can be as effective as statins in reducing LDL-cholesterol. In this controlled study, people eating a low-fat diet with cholesterol-lowering foods such as oat bran and cereal, soy drinks and foods, roasted almonds, and margarine containing plant sterols reduced LDL-C levels 29 percent. Another group taking 20 mg of lovastatin obtained LDL-C reductions of 31 percent, virtually the same. Both approaches also reduced C-reactive protein significantly.[3]

"I am not into statin bashing; heart disease is real and these drugs are saving lives every day," lead author Dr. David Jenkins told *UPI Science*. "What I want to do is simply raise the question, again and again, of what should be the initial therapeutic approach to high LDL-cholesterol for anyone. This study confirms that the answer is, simply, a change in diet."[4]

"Managing diet is the key to treating all common lipid disorders," Dr. James Anderson, professor of medicine and clinical nutrition at the University of Kentucky in Lexington, stated in an accompanying editorial.

"These results are potentially important, given the expense, safety concerns, and intolerance related to statin use."[5]

More and more people are recognizing this and making changes in their diets, and manufacturers are responding with more healthful products (and a lot of junk products too). Overall, we have a long way to go. Just as with doctors' selections of prescription drugs, people's selections of foods are often more greatly influenced by intensive marketing than by medical science or common sense. Doctors say that many of their patients do not want to hear about changing their diets and would rather just pop a pill.

Although pills may reduce cholesterol levels, they do not correct the imbalances in people's systems that cause elevated cholesterol or CRP in the first place. Statins reduce cardiovascular risk about 30 percent, which is good, but it is far from 100 percent. People on statins still have a considerable risk of cardiovascular disease. Reducing cholesterol levels with statins is not the same as healing the system.

Even for people interested in healthier diets, it is less clear today than a decade ago what a healthy diet actually is. Ten years ago there was no doubt: a heart-healthy diet was a low-fat diet. Now this isn't so certain. Low-carb diets have replaced low-fat ones as the new rage, different doctors advocate diametrically opposite approaches, different studies spew out conflicting results, and no one is quite sure what really works for whom. This ferment has its positive side and will undoubtedly lead to greater understanding and better methods, but for now it is creating a lot of confusion.

Still, there are ways to identify the diet that is best for helping you maintain health and lower your risk of cardiovascular disease.

THE GREAT DEBATE: FATS VERSUS CARBOHYDRATES

The crux of the debate raging today centers on whether a low-fat or a low-carbohydrate diet is best for reducing atherosclerosis and cardiovascular disease. In one corner we have Dr. Dean Ornish, the Pritikin Foundation, and the American Heart Association, which advocate low-fat diets. In the other corner, the Dr. Atkins advocates and many others who extol low-carbohydrate, high-fat diets. The debate is intense and important, yet to some degree it is absurd. The fact is, some fats are good and others are bad, and some carbohydrates are good and others are bad—and for most people, health depends more on choosing good fats and good carbohydrates than on strictly adhering to a rigid low-fat or low-carb doctrine.

Moreover, no one diet works for everyone. As with drugs, individual variation is the critical factor with nutrition. Low-fat and low-carb diets can work, but the key question is: Which diet works for you? A doctor recently told me, "My friend went on the Atkins, high-fat diet, and her cholesterol levels came way down. I went on the same diet, and my cholesterol levels went through the roof. Obviously, our systems work differently."

But the diet controversy makes good copy, sells millions of newspapers and magazines, and provides dynamic drama for television, so expect to hear plenty more from the Atkins and Ornish camps and anyone else with a study or opinion. It is interesting to hear these ideas, but always remember that as convincing as someone or some study may sound, it always comes down to your body type and tendencies.

It also ultimately comes down to calories. Whether you are on a low-fat or low-carb diet, if you eat too many calories, it will fail. You will gain weight, and your risk of heart attacks and strokes, as well as of diabetes and high blood pressure, will rise. "There is no magic combination of fat versus carbs versus protein," Dr. Alice Lichtenstein, a nutrition expert at Tufts University, told the *Associated Press* in 2002. "The bottom line is calories, calories, calories."[6] Actually, although I agree with her about calories, it does matter whether you choose a low-fat or low-carb diet. And there are ways of deciding which is best for you.

Low-Fat Diets (Ornish, Pritikin)

Atherosclerosis is infrequently hereditary in origin.
Most of us get atherosclerosis because we consume
too much fat, cholesterol, and calories.[7]
—Dr. W.C.Roberts, *American Journal of Cardiology*

In 1971, when I was a medical intern, I learned that my cholesterol was 265. I shouldn't have been surprised, because my mother's family runs elevated cholesterol levels of 250 to 350 mg/dl, with too much of the bad LDL-C and too little of the good HDL-C. Since then, I have tried many diets. The Pritikin diet worked best, but it only reduced my cholesterol to 215—still too high. A doctor once recommended prescription drugs, but I declined. This was before statins, which I might have taken, but the drug he recommended was Lopid (gemfi-brozil), and I was not impressed with its studies then. The studies showed that Lopid reduced cardiovascular death, but not overall death, so what was the point? Besides, although heart attacks and strokes killed most of my elderly relatives, they usually lived into their 70s or 80s, so I had time to try other things.

During the 1990s I developed a disabling vascular disorder and tried many things to get better. One of them was a vegetarian diet. I was not thinking about my cholesterol level then; I had more immediate problems. Eight months later, when I had some blood tests done, my cholesterol level was 165. I was shocked. I did not know that any diet could reduce cholesterol that much. For eight years, with a modified vegetarian, low-fat diet, I have been able to keep my total cholesterol level in the 160 to 180 mg/dl range. People with family histories like mine are usually told that their cholesterol problems are genetic and that only prescription drugs will work. But "genetic" may not mean "impossible to do anything about." My genetic cholesterol disorder seemed intract-able, but it actually meant that I simply could not handle bad fats. When I eat even small amounts of saturated or hydrogenated fats, my cholesterol and LDL-C levels skyrocket. Yet if I am a hawk about avoiding bad fats, my body does not become a cholesterol-manufacturing machine, and my cholesterol levels stay low.

This is not much different than the 40-percent reductions in LDL-C reported with the low-fat diet rec-ommended by Dr. Dean Ornish, head of the Preventive Medicine Research Institute in Sausalito. "Most people can accomplish comparable reductions in LDL [to statins] by diet and lifestyle alone," stated Dr. Ornish.[8] One of the keys to the success of this approach is getting ample protein. When doing so, people report high levels of satiation and little problem with hunger.[9]

The extensive research on the heart-healthy Mediterranean diet demonstrates the same thing: cholesterol problems are not due to the amount of fats people eat, but the types of fats. Italians and Greeks eat as much fat as Americans, but theirs is primarily olive oil, which provides large amounts of heart-healthy monounsaturated fats. Olive oil also contains phenols that are similar to those found in green tea and red wine that inhibit LDL-C oxidation.[10] Thus, a 2003 study in the *New England Journal of Medicine* reported: "Greater adherence to the traditional Mediterranean diet is associated with a significant reduction in total mortality."[11]

The diet of the people of Okinawa, who have the longest life spans on the planet, contains high amounts of fat (from fish and soy) and carbohydrates (from vegetables and rice), but is low in saturated fats. Eskimos live on very high-fat foods, but Eskimos have low incidences of heart disease and arthritis because the fats they eat are very rich in omega-3 fatty acids.

The lesson is that Atkins, who said, "All fats are good," was wrong. Good fats are good, and bad fats are bad. Americans consume large quantities of bad fats—saturated fats and hydrogenated oils—that elevate cholesterol levels and cause cardiovascular disease. Indeed, every society that has adopted Western dietary habits has suffered major increases in heart attacks and strokes.

The trans fats, the "partially hydrogenated" oils so

prevalent in processed foods, are a special problem. Dr. Walter Willett, one of America's foremost nutrition experts and a professor at the Harvard School of Public Health, states:

Trans fats seem to be uniquely bad because they both raise LDL cholesterol, reduce HDL cholesterol, and also elevate lipoprotein A. There is no other type of fat that has that combination of adverse effects. Some people say that trans fats are only a small percentage of the diet, they are only on average 2–3% of the American diet. But there is no other artificial chemical in our food supply that comes anywhere near that level, and this level of intake could account for. . . 30,000 deaths a year. That is not a trivial number of premature deaths, and they are quite unnecessary.[12]

Margarine was created as a better alternative to saturated-fat-laden butter. If margarines had been marketed in liquid form, allowing their oils to remain unsaturated, they might have been healthful. But in hardening the oils through hydrogenation so they would have the same consistency of butter, trans fatty acids were formed, and it has taken decades to learn that these are more destructive than the saturated fat they were designed to replace. Finally, to warn people about the dangers of trans fatty acids, the FDA now requires trans fats to be listed separately on food labels. The food industry resisted, of course, to their shame.

Advocates of low-fat diets with moderate amounts of protein and high-quality complex carbohydrates have plenty of evidence supporting their perspective. Studies repeatedly show that when people stick with low-fat diets, incidences of coronary disorders, heart attacks, and cardiac deaths plummet. Dr. Caldwell Esselstyn of the Cleveland Clinic reminds us that "although coronary artery disease is the leading killer of men and women in the USA, it is rarely encountered in cultures that base their nutrition primarily on grains, legumes, lentils, vegetables, and fruit."[13] In other words, the doctor is advocating a low-fat, moderate-protein— high-quality—diet based on natural foods. Dr. Dean Ornish has clearly demonstrated that for people with advanced coronary disease, strict restriction of fat, especially saturated and hydrogenated fat, can halt and sometimes reverse atherosclerosis.[14,15]

A low-fat, high-quality diet does not mean going crazy on carbohydrates. It does not mean you can eat unlimited amounts of "low-fat" foods filled with sugars and calories. It does not mean breads and pastries made from refined white flour or loaded with sugar. Bad carbohydrates are just as bad as bad fats. You must select your carbohydrates just as carefully as you select fats.

Most people do not have to adopt austere low-fat diets to obtain heart-healthy results. Good fats, particularly olive oil and adequate omega-3 oils, are healthful. For cooking, use olive oils or canola oil. Dr. Joe Mercola prefers coconut oil to canola, because coconut oil, although a saturated fat, has medicinal properties and does not break down with intense heat.

Good protein means fish, chicken and white meat turkey, lean red meats, soy, beans, and egg whites. Protein and fat are additionally important because they are metabolized more slowly than carbohydrates, so they provide a sense of satiation that lasts many hours after meals. Meals with too few fats and proteins and too many carbohydrates, especially simple carbs like sugars and refined grains, can cause a return of hunger within a few hours after eating—and can raise insulin, triglyceride, and small particle LDL-C levels.

Low-Carbohydrate, High-Fat Diets (Atkins)

Advocates of low-carb, high-fat diets are correct in saying that when people, worried about eating too much fat, switch to low-fat and nonfat foods with more sugar and calories, they do themselves more harm than good. They are correct that too little fat in meals leads to less satiation and rebound hunger. But they are dead wrong when they go to the opposite extreme and claim that all carbohydrates, including complex carbohydrates filled with antioxidants and cancer-preventing substances, are bad and that saturated fat-laden meats, cream sauces, and lard are good. Yet, the low-carb, high-fat fad continues to be praised, and many people think they are eating healthfully when they frequent restaurants offering fat-laden fare. This trend will take us back to the 1950s, when similar diets triggered an epidemic of heart attacks and strokes.

Some people can handle low-carb, high-fat diets, but not high-carb diets. A high intake of poor-quality carbohydrates leads to elevated levels of glucose, insulin, and triglycerides, and reduced levels of HDL-C—a destructive constellation known as metabolic syndrome (or syndrome X). The tendency toward metabolic syndrome is genetically determined. Metabolic syndrome has been recognized by integrative physicians for years and is finally being recognized by mainstream medicine.

This recognition has followed several decades, during which concerns about fats led manufacturers to produce and people to eat foods filled with simple, nutrient-deficient carbohydrates—sugars and white flour—with more calories than the foods they replaced. The result is that since the 1980s, we have seen burgeoning increases in obesity and obesity-related illnesses such as diabetes and high blood pressure. From the 1970s to 1999, obesity increased from 15 percent to 27 percent in the U.S. Today, more than 30 percent of Americans are obese and nearly two-thirds are overweight. The most common culprit: bad carbohydrates—but not all carbohydrates.

Metabolic syndrome is characterized by reduced insulin sensitivity, which is also known as insulin resistance: the inability of a person's cells to respond properly to the insulin that is secreted by the pancreas in response to the carbohydrates eaten. People with normal insulin sensitivity can metabolize carbohydrates properly. When insulin sensitivity is reduced, cells are less able to utilize glucose, and blood glucose levels rise. To compensate, more insulin is produced, but the tissues can become even more insulin resistant, and more and more carbohydrate is converted into fat. People become overweight or obese, which worsens the process. By eating properly and not becoming overweight, many people with a genetic tendency toward metabolic syndrome can avoid the development of the syndrome.

Prevention is key, because the progression of metabolic syndrome leads to its typical features: abdominal obesity, elevated triglycerides, low HDL-C, elevated blood pressure, and an elevated fasting blood glucose level. This is serious: metabolic syndrome is associated with a five- to nine-fold increased risk of diabetes and a two- to three-fold increased risk of cardiovascular mortality.[16] This is why Dr. Jonathan Wright recommends: "If you have type 2 diabetes or symptoms of low blood sugar, or if these problems are in your family, then a low-carb diet probably is your best choice."[17]

About 23 percent of the population has metabolic syndrome.[18] In a recent survey of 60 year olds, 42 percent had diagnosable metabolic syndromes.[19] Integrative practitioners report even higher percentages in their practices. "About 80 percent of the patients I see have metabolic syndrome," Dr. Ron Hoffman, former president of the American College for the Advancement of Medicine, told me. "Of course, my population may be skewed by the kinds of people who decide to see me."[20]

"I see a lot of metabolic syndrome patients," says Jeffrey Baker, MD. "Insulin plays a big role in the elevated cholesterol of many of my patients. Controlling excess carbohydrates is key. The diet I recommend includes clean, lean protein including some meats, avoidance of simple sugars and simple carbohydrates, and moderate exercise."[21]

Dr. Baker makes the key distinction between simple and complex carbohydrates. Simple carbohydrates are quickly converted to glucose and cause quick spikes in insulin levels. Simple carbohydrates include not only sugar and honey, but also potatoes, white rice, and the refined wheat or corn flour found in most breads, crackers, pasta, tortillas, and snacks. Flour, even enriched flour, is quickly broken down into simple sugars and acts just like them. People with metabolic syndrome can eat fruits, but only in moderation because of their high content of fructose, a simple sugar. But fruit is far better than a candy bar or a muffin. Fruit juices are taboo, just as any sweetened beverages are for people with metabolic syndrome. Low-carb foods that are high in alcohols allow manufacturers to claim "low net carbohydrates," but are also discouraged because alcohols are handled pretty much like carbohydrates by the body.

Results with low-carb diets can sometimes be dramatic. An integrative doctor told me of an overweight, middle-aged man with a cholesterol level above 250, and triglyceride and blood glucose levels sky high above 400 and 300, respectively—a classic metabolic syndrome. In fact, these numbers were an improvement: they were worse before the man's mainstream doctor placed him on a statin, and Lopid (to lower triglycerides), and a diabetes drug. The integrative doctor, who is also a board-certified internist, analyzed the man's diet, which contained a lot of refined grains and tons of pasta. By limiting the refined grains and modestly increasing the protein and good oils, the man's blood studies returned to normal within months and he was able to discontinue the drugs.

This is an extreme case, of course, and unless you have diabetes or metabolic syndrome, or tendencies toward these, you do not have to adopt an austere low-carb diet to maintain health. This is why I cringed when I heard Dr. Atkins say flatly, "Fats are good, carbohydrates are bad." Lard is not healthy. Highly saturated fats are not healthy. There may be some people who can handle bad fats, but not the majority and certainly not in their everyday diets. And although some people using the Atkins diet do not get elevations in their cholesterol levels, this does not mean that this diet is healthy in the long run.

The effects of the Atkins diet were underscored in two studies.[22,23] In the studies, people on the Atkins diet for six months lost more weight than those on a low-fat diet. This may be because the high-fat diet worked better, but it may also be because there is a greater initial loss of water from people's tissues with the Atkins diet—a loss that returns later, because at twelve months, the difference in the two diets was insignificant. The media, as expected, trumpeted the better short-term weight loss with the Atkins diet and the better HDL-C and triglyceride numbers in Atkins dieters. But it conveniently overlooked the fact that LDL-C levels did not drop in the Atkins group, yet did drop in the low-fat group. And there were other concerns with the Atkins diet, as one of the studies described:

> The low-carbohydrate diet [Atkins diet] was associated with a greater improvement in some risk factors for coronary heart disease (serum triglycerides and serum HDL cholesterol), but not others (blood pressure, insulin sensitivity, and serum LDL cholesterol). It is also possible that the large amount of saturated fats and small amounts of fruits, vegetables, and fiber consumed during the low-carbohydrate diet can independently increase the risk of coronary heart disease.[23]

I do credit Dr. Atkins for sticking to his guns under

intense criticism in order to make two important points. First, some people do not do well on low-fat diets. Carbohydrate addiction is a reality for some people. Meals should include high-quality fat and protein. Second, some fat is necessary for a lasting sense of satiation after meals, thereby turning off the hunger signal and allowing people to snack less and reduce overall calories. In this vein, the recent studies on the Atkins diet showed that it worked not because it altered people's metabolism, as Atkins thought, but because people simply ate fewer calories.

It is also important to note that in the long-term maintenance phase of the Atkins diet, vegetables are encouraged. Indeed, the Atkins people adjusted their guidelines to include more vegetables. That is because vegetables, with their complex carbohydrates and antioxidants, remain a cornerstone of any healthy diet and can fill you up with relatively few calories. And the fact is, the single most important thing that people with a genetic predisposition toward metabolic syndrome can do is to maintain a healthy weight. The single most important treatment for overweight people with metabolic syndrome is losing weight.

One of the best ways to lose weight is to get more bang for your calories. *The Wall Street Journal* article "The Diet That Works" listed many practical strategies for losing weight. One of the best was to "eat big food," foods that provide a lot of volume for their calories.[24] People tend to eat the same volume of food each day, and soups, vegetables, and fruits provide the greatest volume for the least calories. In contrast, the article noted that a single soda contains 150 calories, which are a lot of calories for the volume. If you normally drink one soda a day, replacing the soda with bottled water every day for a year can produce a loss of 15 pounds. (For every 10 calories you cut every day for a year, you will lose one pound.)

The fad toward fats and away from carbohydrates has given vegetables like carrots a bad rap, because they measure poorly on a scale known as the glycemic index. This index was developed to measure the impact of a food on insulin levels. Unfortunately, the methodology of the glycemic index is flawed, and newer studies using the glycemic load scale reveal that carrots, as well as whole fruits (apples, pears, peaches, berries, etc.), are indeed healthful.[25] Yet, some experts still use the outdated glycemic index and arrive at questionable results. "If you look at tables of glycemic index, you will see things that should bother an intelligent person," states Dr. Gabe Mirkin. "A carrot has almost the same glycemic index as sugar does. This is ridiculous. A carrot is far safer for diabetics than table sugar."[26] Tables listing the glycemic load of common foods can be found at the websites of *Consumer Reports* and the Harvard Medical School. A very complete list was published in the *American Journal of Clinical Nutrition* in 2002 (volume 76, pages 5–56).

Moreover, foods must be considered in the context of the other foods with which they are eaten. Pasta is a high glycemic-load food, but this is partially mitigated when pasta is eaten with olive oil-rich sauces and a salad full of complex carbohydrates. The greater problem by far is the plethora of sodas, candies, sugars, and refined-flour breads, pastries, pancakes, doughnuts, and crackers that are eaten alone or with other refined carbo-hydrate products. The morning doughnut-and-coffee-with-sugar routine is a typical, harmful refined-carbohydrate fix that drives insulin levels up and con-tributes to the metabolic syndrome phenomenon.

GRAINS: THE WHOLE STORY

Recent epidemiological data indicate that diets rich in high-fiber whole grains are associated with lower risk of coronary heart disease (CHD) and type 2 [adult onset] diabetes mellitus. These data are consistent with results from recent metabolic experiments suggesting favorable lipid profiles and glycemic control associated with higher intake of whole grains, but not with refined grains. It seems prudent, therefore, to distinguish whole-grain rather than refined-grain cereal products for the prevention of chronic diseases.[27]

—*Journal of the American College of Nutrition*

Some low-carb, high-fat advocates warn people against eating any types of grains, which are a carbohydrate-rich food. Their warnings might be appropriate for peo-ple with diabetes, but not for most people. The problem with breads and pasta today is not that they are grains, but that 95 percent of them are refined instead of whole grains. Other anti-grain advocates claim that people do best on the foods on which the human species evolved through the eons, and they tout the Neanderthal diet. This does not include grains, which only became part of the human diet around 3,000 BC, so grains just cannot be good. But just because something is new does not mean it is bad. Sanitation, electricity, and temperature-controlled homes were not part of our natural heritage either, but I tend to believe they are changes for the better. So are whole grains.

Some warn that grains are bad because many people cannot handle the gluten contained in wheat. This is true for some people, and an elimination diet to identify food intolerances to gluten-containing grains such as wheat (including durum, semolina, spelt, kamut), rye, barley, and oats has merit for people with chronic disorders. However, rice and corn do not contain gluten and needn't be avoided, nor do buckwheat, millet, amaranth, soy, or teff flours.

Other grain foes argue that grains have a high glycemic index and are quickly digested into glucose, pushing blood glucose levels and insulin production way up, producing metabolic syndrome. But not everyone is prone to metabolic syndrome, and although refined grains may catapult insulin levels, whole grains don't. An article in the *American Journal of Clinical Nutrition* explained:

> During the past decade, several lines of evidence have collectively provided strong support for a relation between diets and diabetes incidence. In diabetic patients, evidence from medium-term studies suggests that replacing high-glycemic-index carbohydrates with low-glycemic-index foods will improve glycemic control and, among persons treated with insulin, will reduce hypoglycemic episodes. These dietary changes, which can be made by replacing products made with white flour and potatoes with whole-grain, minimally refined cereal products, have

also been associated with a lower risk of cardiovascular disease and can be an appropriate component of recommendations for an overall healthy diet.[28]

As demonstrated in the inset on pages 100–101, study after study has proven that whole grains are associated with less cardiovascular disease and diabetes. Refined grains are quickly digested and impact the body like sugars, but whole grains, with their complex structures and high concentrations of fiber, protein, and antioxidants, are digested much more slowly. Refined grains cause insulin levels to spike; whole grains don't.

One of the latest studies, from Boston's Brigham and Women's Hospital and the Harvard Medical School, was published in the *American Journal of Clinical Nutrition.* This was a prospective study, which is one of the most powerful types of clinical studies, following 86,190 male doctors for five years. Comparing matched groups that differed only in their intake of refined versus whole grains, the study found:

> Both total mortality and cardiovascular disease mortality-specific mortality were inversely associated with whole-grain but not refined-grain breakfast cereal intake. These prospective data highlight the importance of distinguishing whole-grain from refined-grain cereals in the prevention of chronic diseases.[34]

Indeed, in an earlier study in the same journal, people who ate cereals, muffins, spaghetti, breads and rolls—and even chocolate chip cookies—made with whole grains had reduced after-meal and fasting insulin levels. Of course, when made with refined grains, these foods cause insulin levels to spike. But in this study, even in overweight subjects, who usually have even greater insulin spiking, the whole-grain foods produced improved insulin response. This study, backed by extensive epidemiologic evidence, showed that there is an "inverse association between consumption of cereal fiber or whole grains and type 2 diabetes, cardiovascular disease, and total mortality."[35]

Just as olive and omega-3 oils have far different effects on human physiology and health than saturated and hydrogenated fats, whole grains have far different effects than refined grains and other simple carbohydrates. Epidemiologic studies involving tens of thousands of people have repeatedly shown reduced risks of heart attacks in people consuming whole grains. Other studies have shown that whole grains reduce cancer risks.

"Whole grains are rich sources of a wide range of phytochemicals with anticarcinogenic properties," Dr. Joanne Slavin, Professor of Food and Nutrition at the University of Minnesota, told *The New York Times.* "Some of these phytochemicals block DNA damage and suppress cancer cell growth."[36] They are also a rich source of minerals that are deficient in many diets. For example, a half cup of white rice contains only 4 milligrams of magnesium, but the same amount of brown rice contains 47 mg. A slice of white bread contains 6 mg of magnesium, yet whole wheat bread contains 24 mg.[37]

The benefits of whole grains are so well proven, the FDA allows food manufacturers to trumpet their benefits on their packaging:

Whole Grains, Diabetes, and Cancer

Here is a small sample of the many articles in the medical literature about the benefits of whole-grain foods.

• *American Journal of Clinical Nutrition:* "Whole grains can provide a substantial contribution to the improvement of the diets of Americans. A number of whole grain foods and grain fiber sources are beneficial in reduction of insulin resistance and improvement in glucose tolerance. Dietary recommendations of health organizations suggest consumption of three servings a day of whole grain foods; however, Americans generally fall below this standard."[29]

• *American Journal of Clinical Nutrition:* "Consistent findings from prospective studies of diverse populations and supporting data from metabolic trials strongly support the premise that an increased intake of whole-grain foods can lower the risk of type 2 diabetes."[30]

• *American Journal of Public Health:* "These findings

Diets rich in whole-grain foods and other plant foods low in total fat, saturated fat and cholesterol, may help reduce the risk of heart disease and certain cancers.[38]

The evidence is overwhelming: whole grains are beneficial for most people. Some diets such as Dr. Mercola's No-Grain Diet recommend avoidance of all grains during the early phases of treatment of carbohydrate addiction. A small percentage of people may be so sensitive to any carbohydrates that grains of any kind are a problem. But for most people, whole grains have suggest that substituting whole- for refined-grain products may decrease the risk of diabetes mellitus."[31]

• *Journal of the American College of Nutrition:* "Dietary guidance recommends consumption of whole grains for the prevention of cancer. Epidemiologic studies find that whole grains are protective against cancer, especially gastrointestinal cancers such as gastric and colonic, and hormonally-dependent cancers including breast and prostate."[32]

• *Nutrition and Metabolism in Cardiovascular Disease:* "Whole grain food intake was consistently related to reduced risk of several types of cancer, particularly of the upper digestive tract neoplasms. Epidemiological evidence of the relation between fiber and colorectal cancer indicate possible protections. In contrast, refined grain intake was associated to increased risk of different types of cancer, pointing to a potential role of insulin-like growth factor 1."[33]

a well-deserved place as one of the cornerstones of a healthy diet.

Whole-grain breads, cereals, and even pasta are so plentiful today, it is easy to find tasty products. But be sure to check the ingredients, because many products boasting "whole grains" are not entirely whole-grained, but in fact contain mostly white flour. Fortunately, food manufacturers are gradually conforming to consumers' demand for fully whole-grain products. It is time for you to replace the refined grains in your diet with whole grains.

WHICH DIET
IS BEST FOR YOU?

It is unfortunate that, while Western science has greatly increased our understanding of human physiology and nutrition in recent decades, our everyday nutrition has become increasingly filled with harmful and unnatural foods that have caused epidemics of obesity, hypercholesterolemia, hypertension and other cardiovascular disease, metabolic syndrome, and diabetes. The origins of this paradox are not hard to discover. During the twentieth century, major changes were made in food production without any consideration for their long-term effects. Western diets veered from natural foods to manufactured products based on shelf life, taste, and salesmanship. Whole grains were replaced with refined grains. Healthy oils were replaced with hydrogenated oils. Sugar use skyrocketed. It was a recipe for disaster.

Our sources of animal protein saw dramatic changes, too. In previous centuries, humans ate animals that grazed on grasses instead of being fattened on grains. When raised on grasses, animals develop high levels of heart-healthy omega-3 oils and less saturated fat. In the twentieth century, we got the saturated fat (and hormones and antibiotics) with little omega-3 oil from our animal products.

Food manufacturers also learned that products filled with fats and sugars taste and smell better and are nearly irresistible. Intensive advertising on television and in the print media lulled us into believing food selection is all about taste, not health. The food industry created and catered to this new taste-fixated market.

The market was us making bad food choices. The results of all of these changes have been obvious since the 1950s, and we have been trying to find our way out ever since. First, low-fat, high-carb diets became the way. Then, the pendulum swung to the other extreme of low-carb, high-fat diets. Such foods will take us right back to the high-fat heart disease epidemics of the mid-twentieth century.

So which is the villain: fats or carbohydrates? My answer is simple:

- Bad fats (saturated and hydrogenated fats) are bad.

- Good fats (olive oil, omega-3 fatty acids, canola oil for cooking) are good.

- Bad carbohydrates (simple sugars, processed flour) are bad.

- Good carbohydrates (complex carbohydrates as in vegetables, fruit, and whole grains) are good.

You do not have to become carbo-phobic or fat-phobic to eat right. Human bodies need fat, carbohydrate, and protein. What is the right balance? Which diet—low-fat or low-carb—is best for you? For most people, the answer lies between the two extremes of Atkins and Ornish: a balanced diet based on healthful foods. Neither an extreme low-fat nor extreme low-carb diet is necessary or desirable for cardiovascular health in most cases. The best diets contain good fats, good carbohydrates, and good protein—lean, clean protein, as Dr. Baker puts it—in a healthful balance. The best diets are based on olive oil, omega-3 oils, vegetables, whole grains, fruit, nuts, legumes, fish, chicken, lean meats, and low-fat or non-fat dairy. These are the pillars of the Mediterranean diet, the DASH diet that has been proven to reduce high blood pressure, and to a large extent the Okinawan diet and the South Beach diet.

Indeed, both the Ornish and Atkins approaches recommend many of these same foods. This really is not surprising, because the foundations of a heart-healthy diet are clear, as described by nationally-recognized experts Drs. Frank Hu and Walter Willett:

> Substantial evidence indicates that diets using non-hydrogenated unsaturated fats as the predominant form of dietary fat, whole grains as the main form of carbohydrates, an abundance of fruits and vegetables, and adequate omega-3 fatty acids can offer significant protection against coronary heart disease. Such diets, together with regular physical activity, avoidance of smoking, and maintenance of a healthy body weight, may prevent the majority of cardiovascular disease in Western populations.[38]

It can be helpful to know whether your metabolism runs better with a higher ratio of fats or carbohydrates. A new method for doing so is metabolic typing. This approach, based on the book *The Metabolic Typing Diet* by Wolcott and Fahey, measures many different factors in determining your physiological and psychological tendencies, and the diet that fits your profile the best.[39] Wolcott's work is based on studies and writings that go back a century. The book offers a test that defines your best diet. Although I think the test requires refinement, the basic tenets of the book are sound, and I agree with

Wolcott's main theme: different people do well on different food balances. Or, in Wolcott's words:

> Standardized nutritional approaches fail to recognize that, for genetic reasons, people are all very different from one another on a biochemical or metabolic level. Due to widely varying hereditary influences, we all process or utilize foods and nutrients very differently. Thus, the very same nutritional protocol that enables one person to lead a long healthy life full of robust health can cause serious illness in someone else. As the ancient Roman philosopher Lucretius once said, 'One man's food is another's poison.' It turns out his statement is quite literally true.[40]

If you have elevated cholesterol, CRP, or other risk factors, you may have to work with a health professional. Because diet is so key to treating these conditions, you should seek a practitioner who understands not only the importance of diet, but also that different people do well with different approaches. Start with a low-fat, low-carb, or a balanced carb-fat-protein diet and monitor its effect on your cholesterol, triglyceride, LDL-C particle size, and glucose levels. If the first diet does not produce the desired results, try another. In this way, it is easy to identify the diet that is best for you. What you eat is either facilitating health or fueling disease. Most people with elevated cholesterol or metabolic syndrome have eaten their way to their disorders. Although I did not know it, I certainly ate my way to my cholesterol problem, and now I have eaten my way out of it. Now I load each meal with several low-calorie, high-volume vegetables, with good oils, protein, whole grains, and a piece of fruit—a diet that allows me to maintain a low cholesterol and proper weight while never feeling hungry.

People repeatedly tell me that they hate taking medication. Most people with high cholesterol, high triglycerides, elevated homocysteine, or metabolic syndrome do not have to take medication. You do not have to become one of the 62 percent of the population who is overweight, or one of the 50 percent of Americans who develop advanced atherosclerosis and coronary symptoms[7], or one of the 90 percent who ultimately develop high blood pressure. You and your children do not have to be among the burgeoning numbers of diabetics.

Identify your metabolic type, adopt the proper diet, orient your meals to high-volume, low-calorie foods, and monitor the results. If a low-fat diet causes problems, add more healthy fats and reduce the carbs, especially the simple carbs. If a low-carb diet causes your cholesterol levels to jump, switch to a low-fat, high complex-carbohydrate approach. Balance these diets with enough protein. Keep your weight down. Some experts believe that it does not really matter which diet you use as long as it helps you maintain a healthy weight. Find the diet that works best for you and stick to it. Commit yourself to it. You only get one body. Treat it like it's important to you.

A LITTLE EXERCISE
MAKES A BIG DIFFERENCE

You already know that exercise is important. You know that our bodies are biologically designed for activity, and that our current culture of inactivity is unnatural.

Indeed, exercise is so important that it is better to be somewhat overweight and exercising than to be at a good weight and not exercising.

"Of all the behaviors that are health related, physical activity is by far the most important," Dr. Tim Byers, professor of preventive medicine at the University of Colorado School of Medicine in Denver and co-chairman of the American Cancer Society's cancer prevention guideline committee, told *USA Today*. "It's strongly protective for heart disease, diabetes and some types of cancer, and regular physical activity is essential for a lifetime of weight control."[41] This is not a minority position. "The best alternative method is exercise, which reduces cardiac mortality 50% (much better than statins) and reduces overall mortality as well," stated Dr. Wayne Anderson, Chairman of Family Practice and the Preventive Health Task Force, Scripps Clinic, at a recent conference.

You do not have to overdo it to obtain benefits from exercise. Studies show that just a little exercise a day is nearly as effective for maintaining health as triathlon training. Thirty to forty-five minutes a day is enough. Yet, fewer than 50 percent of Americans get thirty minutes of exercise a day. The most common excuse is, "I can't find the time to exercise." No doubt, with so many people working fifty to sixty hours a week these days, it is difficult. Here is a suggestion if you cannot find the time to exercise: get a treadmill or exercise bike, place it in your den and use it in the evening when you watch television or read. By combining exercise with other routine activities, it does not take any extra time from other obligations, and exercise passes quickly while watching TV or a movie. If you are older or have medical problems, check with your doctor before starting an exercise regimen.

Start gradually in order to avoid quick burnout. Don't push it. It is better to exercise at a low, comfortable intensity for thirty to sixty minutes than at high intensity for short, unpleasant durations. You will enjoy it more, and with consistency your strength and endurance will increase naturally and make more strenuous workouts easy. Surprisingly quickly, exercise will make you feel stronger, healthier, fit, better in every way.

YOUR RIGHT OF INFORMED CONSENT INCLUDES ALTERNATIVE THERAPIES

For millions of people, the first symptom of heart disease is a heart attack. Heart disease and stroke remain our number 1 and number 3 leading killers. Although these diseases may strike suddenly, they take decades to develop. You do not want to wait until they occur before getting serious about maintaining cardiovascular health. Atherosclerosis may be a slowly developing disease, but once entrenched it is difficult to stop and even more difficult to reverse.

An ounce of prevention is better than any amount of cure, because with cardiovascular disease, nothing matches prevention. Prevention begins with wise decisions made as early in life as possible. I would like to see every young person have a complete blood analysis that includes cholesterol levels, C-reactive protein, triglycerides, and homocysteine. Knowing where you stand is essential for knowing what to do.

The most effective preventatives for cardiovascular disease are a healthful diet, maintaining an ideal weight, exercising regularly, and not smoking. Even with these healthy habits, some people will develop elevated LDL-C or low HDL-C. Others will have a high homocysteine level or a genetic predisposition to small particle LDL-C or lipoprotein A. Treating these conditions is not usually an emergency. Except for people with severe cardiovascular disorders, there is time to make informed decisions. The treatment of cardiovascular risk factors requires a life-long effort. It is a marathon, not a sprint, so it is important for you to feel good about the methods you adopt.

Many doctors are most comfortable with using statin drugs, but many patients are not thrilled with the idea of taking a powerful and expensive prescription drug for the rest of their lives. (See page 112 for a comparison of costs of prescription drugs and natural supplements.) Many people accept statin therapy because this is what their doctors recommend and because they are not told about the alternatives. Cardiologist William Davis states, "It may be better to regard statin therapy as a solution only after other natural alternatives have been exhausted. The problem is that many people are unaware of many of the strategies that work."[1]

Before your doctor prescribes a statin drug, you have a right to be informed about the effective natural therapies for reducing cholesterol or other cardiovascular risk factors. This right is known as informed consent. The American Medical Association's Code of Medical Ethics defines informed consent as follows:

> The patient's right of self-decision can be effectively exercised only if the patient possesses enough information to enable an intelligent choice.... The physician has an ethical obligation to help the patient make choices from among the therapeutic alternatives consistent with good medical practice.[2]

The natural cholesterol-reducing therapies discussed in this book are, according to the AMA definition, "therapeutic alternatives consistent with good medical practice," so you have a right to be informed about them. It is not enough for patients to be offered statin drugs as the only solution. Most people with elevated LDL-C fall into low or moderate risk categories, and most of them can reach their treatment goals with a heart-healthy diet and a natural alternative therapy. And they have a right to know this.

Unfortunately, our healthcare system does not have a good track record of providing informed consent when medications are prescribed. Informed consent is always provided before people undergo surgery, but it is infrequently provided before people receive prescription drugs. In one study of interactions between doctors and patients in doctors' offices, fewer than 10 percent of the patients received enough information to fulfill their rights of informed consent.[3]

TOWARD CREATING A TRULY INTEGRATIVE HEALTHCARE SYSTEM

One reason why informed consent is rarely provided is that most doctors know little about the many natural alternatives for reducing cholesterol. This is the reality of the mainstream healthcare system today. You can help. Tell your doctor about the proven-effective alternatives or show him or her this book. Help spread the word. Your doctor is not going to hear about effective natural alternatives from drug company sales reps, drug advertising, drug company-designed studies published in medical journals, or drug company-subsidized semi-

Table 7.1. Natural Supplements Cost Less

Natural cholesterol-lowering supplements cost much less than many prescription drugs. Costs of natural supplements reflect prices listed in May 2005. The prices of these natural supplements may be a bit higher than some generic products sold in health food stores and on the Internet. Studies have shown that some supplements do not contain the amounts claimed on their labels, so I recommend products from well-known companies with good quality control programs. However, if cost is an issue, you can start with a cheaper generic product and see if it lowers your cholesterol levels adequately. Prescription prices are from the Costco pharmacy website, January 2005 (Costco pharmacy prices are often much lower than those at local pharmacies).

Product	Monthly Cost
CHOLESTEROL-LOWERING AGENTS	
Prescription Statin Medications	
Lipitor 20 mg	$96
Pravachol 40 mg	$126
Zocor 40 mg	$123
Generic Lovastatin (same as Mevacor) 20 mg	$19
Over-the-Counter Natural Alternatives	
Red Yeast Rice 600 mg	$10–$20
Plant Sterols 600 mg	$10
Policosanol	$15–$30
INTERMEDIATE-ACTING NIACIN COMPOUNDS	
Prescription	
Niaspan 1,000 mg	$60–$120
Over-The-Counter	
Inositol Hexaniacinate 500 mg	$12–$36

nars and meetings. The drug industry has long known that if it dominates the information that doctors receive, it can greatly influence the decisions that doctors make. That is why the drug companies spend more than $15,000 annually on marketing to each American doctor. The strategy works and is not likely to change any time soon. This is why you must take an active role in helping to keep your doctors current about the issues and options that concern you.

In a rational healthcare system, solutions for most disorders would begin with nutrition, then natural interventions, and then pharmaceuticals. The problem is, in today's medical-pharmaceutical complex, doctors are taught to trust pharmaceuticals above all else, and drugs are usually the first solution rather than the last. Even when we discover the underlying mechanism of a disease, the research money does not go to discovering a nutritional or natural solution. The money goes to finding a patentable, profitable, synthetic solution—a drug. Because the drug is not a natural product, it will cause side effects. Nevertheless, when the new drug receives FDA approval, the media jumps on board, headlines abound, intensive marketing toward doctors and consumers is launched—is it any wonder why we are a drug-oriented society?

The result is that today we have a medical system that is divided into two camps, mainstream and alternative. We have hundreds of thousands of mainstream doctors who know about medications, and we have a few thousand alternative doctors who know about natural therapies. In an ideal system, all doctors would be integrative doctors, combining the best of both worlds.

You shouldn't have to go to two doctors to get one full picture. All doctors should be knowledgeable about the full range of therapies for elevated cholesterol and CRP, as well as for everything else they treat. But this is not the reality today.

My purpose in writing this book is to provide good information based on scientific study and clinical experience about the natural, effective therapies for improving cardiovascular risk factors and for promoting heart health. One of my goals is to help readers obtain the best and safest treatments. Another goal is to provide an objective source of quality information in order to help bring the healthcare system a step closer to becoming fully integrative in its methods. Prescription statin drugs have their uses, especially for people with advanced cardiovascular disease, but for the great majority of people with elevated cholesterol or other risk factors, the natural therapies deserve consideration. The only doctors who can provide patients with fully informed consent are those who possess a good grasp of both the prescription and natural treatment choices.

If, by reading this book, you now know about the many natural therapies available for reducing cholesterol or other cardiovascular risk factors, you can inform your doctor and, together, discuss all of the treatment possibilities. Enabling such discussions between readers and their doctors has been my ultimate goal in writing this book.

REFERENCES

Chapter 1

1. "Achieving a Heart-Healthy and Stroke-Free Nation: The Burden of Heart Disease and Stroke in the United States." U.S. Department of Health and Human Services, accessed May 10, 2004:www. healthierus.gov/steps/summit/prevportfolio/strategies/reducing/heart/burden.htm.

2. Davis, W. "Cholesterol & Statin Drugs: separating hype from reality." *Life Extension Magazine,* Collector's Edition, Mar. 2005:114–124.

3. Parker-Pope, T. "Breakthrough! Ten major medical advances you're likely to see in the coming year." *The Wall Street Journal,* Jan. 26, 2004:R1.

4. Gandhi, TK, Burstin, HR, Cook, EF, et al. "Drug complications in outpatients." *Journal of General Internal Medicine* 2000;15:149–154.

5. Jackevicius, CA, Mamdani, M, Tu, JV. "Adherence with statin therapy in elderly patients with and without acute coronary syndromes." *JAMA* 2002;288:462–467.

6. Benner, JS, Glynn, RJ, Mogun, H, et al. "Long-term persistence in use of statin therapy in elderly patients." *JAMA* 2002;288:455–461.

Chapter 2

1. Simopoulos, AP, Robinson, J. *The Omega Diet.* 1999:HarperCollins, New York.

2. Roberts, WC. "Getting more people on statins." *American Journal of Cardiology* 2002;9:683–685.

3. Sacks, FM, Pfeffer, MA, Moye, LA, et al. "The effect of pravastatin on coronary events after myocardial infarction in patients with

average cholesterol levels." Cholesterol and Recurrent Events Trial investigators. *New England Journal of Medicine* 1996;335(14):1001–9.

4. Shepherd, J, Cobbe, SM, Ford, I, et al. "Prevention of coronary heart disease with pravastatin in men with hypercholesterolemia." West of Scotland Coronary Prevention Study Group. *New England Journal of Medicine* 1995;333(20):1301–7.

5. Downs, JR, Clearfield, M, Weis, S, et al. "Primary prevention of acute coronary events with lovastatin in men and women with average cholesterol levels: results of AFCAPS/TexCAPS." Air Force/Texas Coronary Atherosclerosis Prevention Study. *JAMA* 1998;279(20):1615–1622.

6. "Randomised trial of cholesterol lowering in 4444 patients with coronary heart disease: the Scandinavian Simvastatin Survival Study (4S)." *Lancet* 1994;344(8934):1383–1389.

7. The Long-Term Intervention with Pravastatin in Ischemic Disease (LIPID) Study Group. "Prevention of cardiovascular events and death with pravastatin in patients with coronary heart disease and a broad range of initial cholesterol levels." *New England Journal of Medicine* 1998;339:1349–1357.

8. Gotto AM Jr. "Lipid management in patients at moderate risk for coronary heart disease: insights from the Air Force/Texas Coronary Atherosclerosis Prevention Study (AFCAPS/TexCAPS)." *American Journal of Medicine* 1999;107(2A):36S-39S.

9. Whitaker, J. "Treatments for Elevated Cholesterol." www.Dr Whitaker.com:10/28/02.

10. Executive Summary of the Third Report of the National Cholesterol Education Program (NCEP) Expert Panel on Detection, Evaluation, and Treatment of High Blood Cholesterol in Adults. *JAMA* 2001;285(19):2486–97.

11. Jacotot, B, Banga, JD, Pfister, P, Mehra, M. "Efficacy of a low dose-range of fluvastatin in the treatment of primary hypercholesterolaemia." *British Journal of Clinical Pharmacology* 1994;38(3):257–63.

12. Gonzalez, ER. "The pharmacist's role in lipid reduction therapy." *Pharmacy Times* 63(4):65–70.

13. American Society of Hospital Pharmacists. *American Hospital Formulary Service, Drug Information 2002.* Gerald K. McEvoy, Editor. Bethesda: 2002.

14. Davis, W. "Cholesterol & Statin Drugs: separating hype from reality." *LEF Magazine,* collector's edition, Mar. 2005:114–124.

15. Ridker, PM, Rifai, N, Rose, L, et al. R. "Comparison of C-reactive protein and low-density lipoprotein cholesterol levels in the prediction of first cardiovascular events." *New England Journal of Medicine* 2002;347:1557–1565.

16. Albert, MA, Glynn, RJ, Ridker, PM. "Plasma concentration of C-reactive protein and the calculated Framingham Coronary Heart Disease Risk Score." *Circulation* 2003;108(2):161–5.

17. Sinatra, S. Statins: grossly overprescribed for cholesterol and underprescribed for internal inflammation. *The Sinatra Health Report,* Sept. 2002;8:1.

18. Grady, D. "Study Says a Protein May Be Better Than Cholesterol in Predicting Heart Disease Risk." *The New York Times;* NYTimes.com:Nov. 14, 2002.

19. Ravnskov, U. "Is atherosclerosis caused by high cholesterol?" *QJM (Quarterly Journal of Medicine)* 2002;95:397–403.

20. Winslow, R. "Study Confirms Better Predictor of Heart Risk." *The Wall Street Journal,* Nov. 14, 2002:B$_1$,3.

21. Walsh, BW, Paul, S, Wild RA, et al. "The Effects of Hormone Replacement Therapy and Raloxifene on C-Reactive Protein and Homocysteine in Healthy Postmenopausal Women: A Randomized, Controlled Trial." *Journal of Clinical Endocrinology and Metabolism* 2004;85:214–218.

22. Simopoulos, AP. "Essential Fatty Acids in Health and Chronic Disease." *American Journal of Clinical Nutrition* 1999;70(suppl):560S-569S.

23. Simopoulos, AP. "The Mediterranean diets: What is so special about the diet of Greece?" *Journal of Nutrition* 2001;131:3065S-3073S.

24. Block, G, Jensen, C, Dietrich, M, et al. "Plasma C-reactive protein concentrations in active and passive smokers: influence of antiox-

idant supplementation." *Journal of the American College of Nutrition* 2004;23:141–147.

25. Ariyo, AA, Thach, C, Tracy, R. "Lp(a) Lipoprotein, Vascular Disease, and Mortality in the Elderly." *New England Journal of Medicine* 2003;349:2108–2115.

26. Saely, CH, Marte, T, Drexel, H. "Lp(a) Lipoprotein, Vascular Disease, and Mortality in the Elderly." *New England Journal of Medicine* 2004;350:1150–1152.

27. Ehmke, J. More reasons to avoid statin drugs: does Lipitor raise lipoprotein A? Dr. Mercola Website, Aug. 13, 2003:www.mercola.com/2003/aug/13/statin_drugs.htm.

28. McCully, KS. "Homocysteine, folate, vitamin B_6, and cardiovascular disease." *JAMA* 1998;280:417.

Chapter 3

1. Cannon, CP, Braunwald, E, McCabe, CH, et al. "Comparison of intensive and moderate lipid lowering with statins after acute coronary syndromes." *New England Journal of Medicine* 2004;350: 1495–1504.

2. Law, ML, Watt, HC, Wald, NJ. "The underlying risk of death after myocardial infarction in the absence of treatment." *Archives of Internal Medicine* 2002;162:2405–2410.

3. Grundy, SM, Cleeman, JI, Bairey, CN, et al. "Implications of recent clinical trials for the National Cholesterol Education Program Adult Treatment Panel III Guidelines." *Circulation* 2004;110:227–239.

Chapter 4

1. Ault, A. U.S. Alternative Medicine Report Spurs Controversy. Reuters Health, Mar. 25, 2002:www.reuters.com.

2. Villarosa, L. "The Verdict Is Still out on Alternative Medicine." *The New York Times,* Apr. 13, 2002:nytimes.com.

3. Heber, D, Lembertas, A, Qy, L, et al. "An analysis of nine proprietary Chinese red yeast rice dietary supplements." *Journal of Alternative and Complementary Medicine* 2001;7:133–39.

4. Morelli, V, Zoorob, RJ. "Congestive Heart Failure and Hypercholesterolemia: Alternative Therapies, Part 2." *American Family Physician* 2000;62:1325–30.

5. Heber, D, Yip, I, Ashley, JM, et al. "Cholesterol-lowering effects of a proprietary Chinese red-yeast-rice dietary supplement." *American Journal of Clinical Nutrition* 1999;69:231–36.

6. Keithley, JK, Swanson, B, Sha, BE, et al. "A pilot study of the safety and efficacy of cholestin in treating HIV-related dyslipidemia." *Nutrition* 2002;18:201–4.

7. Patrick, L, Uzick, M. "Cardiovascular disease: C-reactive protein and the inflammatory disease paradigm." *Alternative Medicine Review* 2001;6:248–271.

8. Schardt, D. "The heart of the matter: some supplements work... others are worthless." *Nutrition Action Health Letter* 2004;31:8–11.

9. Executive Summary of the Third Report of the National Cholesterol Education Program (NCEP) Expert Panel on Detection, Evaluation, and Treatment of High Blood Cholesterol in Adults. *JAMA* 2001;285(19):2486–97.

10. Whitaker, J. *Slash your cholesterol in 30 days without drugs.* Potomac, MD: Phillips Health, 2002.

11. McKenney, J. "New perspectives on the use of niacin in the treatment of lipid disorders." *Archives of Internal Medicine* 2004;164: 697–705.

12. American Society of Hospital Pharmacists. *American Hospital Formulary Service, Drug Information 2002.* Gerald K. McEvoy, Editor. Bethesda: 2002.

13. *Physicians' Desk Reference,* 54th Edition. Montvale, N.J.: Medical Economics Company, 2000.

14. Head, KA. "Inositol Hexaniacinate: a Safer Alternative to Niacin." *Alternative Medicine Review* 1996;1:176–184.

15. Inositol Hexaniacinate. *Alternative Medicine Review* 1998;3: 222–23.

16. Sinatra, S. "Statins: grossly overprescribed for cholesterol and

underprescribed for internal inflammation." *The Sinatra Health Report,* Sept. 2002;8:1.

17. Gouni-Berthold, I, Berthold, HK. "Policosanol: Clinical Pharmacology and Therapeutic Significance of a New Lipid-Lowering Agent." *American Heart Journal* 2002;143:356–65.

18. Pons, P, Mas, R, Illnait, J, et al. "Efficacy and safety of policosanol in patients with primary hypercholesterolemia." *Current Therapeutics and Research* 1992;52:507–513.

19. Aneros, E, Mas, R, Calderon, B, et al. "Effect of policosanol in lowering cholesterol levels in patients with type 2 hypercholesterolemia." *Current Therapeutics and Research* 1995;56:176–182.

20. Aneros, E, Calderon, B, Mas, R, et al. "Effect of successive dose increases of policosanol on the lipid profile and tolerability of treatment." *Current Therapeutics and Research* 1993:54:304–312.

21. Castano, G, Mas, R, Fernandez, L, et al. "Effects of policosanol 20 versus 40 mg/day in the treatment of patients with type II hypercholesterolemia: a 6-month double-blind study." *International Journal Of Clinical Pharmacologic Research* 2001;21:43–57.

22. Ortensi, G, Gladstein, J, Valli, H, et al. "A comparative study of policosanol versus simvastatin in elderly patients with hypercholesterolemia." *Current Therapeutics and Research* 1997;58:390–401.

23. Castano, G, Mas, R, Fernandez, L, et al. "Efficacy and tolerability of policosanol compared with lovastatin in patients with type 2 hypercholesterolemia and concomitant coronary risk factors." *Current Therapeutics and Research* 2000;61:137–146.

24. Janikula, M. "Policosanol: a new treatment for cardiovascular disease?" *Alternative Medicine* Review 2002;7:203–217.

25. Jones, P. Plant sterols. Designs For Health Seminar, Apr. 27, 2005.

26. Chagan, L, Ioselovich, A, Asherova, L, Cheng, JW. "Use of alternative pharmacotherapy in management of cardiovascular diseases." *American Journal of Managed Care* 2002;8(3):270–85.

27. Lichtenstein, AH. "Plant sterols and blood lipid levels." *Current Opinion in Clinical Nutrition and Metabolic Care* 2002;5(2):147–52.

28. Moghadasian, MH, Frohlich, JJ. "Effects of dietary phytosterols on cholesterol metabolism and atherosclerosis: clinical and experimental evidence." *American Journal of Medicine* 1999;107:588–594.

29. Kerckhoffs, DA, Brouns, F, Hornstra, G, Mensink, RP. "Effects on the Human Serum Lipoprotein Profile of beta-Glucan, Soy Protein and Isoflavones, Plant Sterols and Stanols, Garlic and Tocotrienols." *Journal of Nutrition* 2002;132(9):2494–2505.

30. Nestelss PJ. "Adulthood treatment: Cholesterol-lowering with plant sterols." *Medical Journal of Australia* 2002;176(11 Suppl):S122. Abstract.

31. Lupton, JR, Turner, ND. "Dietary fiber and coronary disease: does the evidence support an association." *Current Atherosclerosis Report* 2003;5:500–505.

32. Weil, A. Cardiovascular disease, June 6, 2003:www.drweil.com.

33. Singh, RB, Niaz, MA, Ghosh, S. "Hypolipidemic and Antioxidant Effects of Commiphora mukul As an Adjunct to Dietary Therapy in Patients with Hypercholesterolemia." *Cardiovascular Drugs and Therapeutics* 1994;8:659–64.

34. Nityanand, S, Srivastava, JS, Asthana, OP. "Clinical Trials of Guggulipid." *Journal of the Association of Physicians of India* 1990;37:323–28.

35. Szapary, PO, Wolfe, ML, Bloedon, LT, et al. "Guggulipid for the Treatment of Hypercholesterolemia: A Randomized Controlled Trial." *JAMA* 2003;290:765–772.

36. Maugh, TH. "Herbal extract is faulted in study." *Los Angeles Times,* Aug. 13, 2003:A9.

37. Szapary, PO. Personal correspondence, Dec. 1, 2003.

38. Silagy, C, Neil, A. "Garlic as a lipid lowering agent—a meta-analysis." *Journal of the Royal College of Physicians London* 1994; 28:39–45.

39. Gardner, CD, Chatterjee, LM, Carlson, JJ. "The effect of a garlic preparation on plasma lipid levels in moderately hypercholesterolemic adults." *Atherosclerosis* 2001;154:213–20.

40. Steiner, M, Khan, AH, Holbert, D, Lin, RI. "A double-blind crossover study in moderately hypercholesterolemic men that compared the effect of aged garlic extract and placebo ministrations on blood lipids." *American Journal of Clinical Nutrition* 1996; 64:866–70.

41. Stevinson, C, Pittler, MH, Ernst, E. "Garlic for treating hypercholesterolemic. A meta-analysis of randomized clinical trials." *Annals of Internal Medicine* 2000;133:420–29.

42. Whitaker, J. Treatments for Elevated Cholesterol, 2002: www.DrWhitaker.com.

43. Food and Drug Administration. Food labeling: health claims; soy protein and coronary heart disease. 21 CFR Part 101. Federal Register 1999;64:57700–57733.

44. Clarkson, TB. "Soy, soy phytoestrogens and cardiovascular disease." *Journal of Nutrition* 2002;132:566S-569S.

45. Tonstad, S, Smerud, K, Hoie, L. "The comparison of the effects of 2 doses of soy protein or casein on serum lipids, serum lipoproteins, and plasma total homocysteine in hypercholesterolemic subjects." *American Journal of Clinical Nutrition* 2002;76:78–84.

46. Desroches, S, Mauger, JF, Ausman, LM, et al. "Soy Protein Favorably Affects LDL Size Independently of Isoflavones in Hypercholesterolemic Men and Women." *Journal of Nutrition* 2004;134: 574–579.

47. Sheehan, D, Doerge, D. Letter to the Food and Drug Administration, Department of Health and Human Services. Feb. 18, 1999.

48. Mercola, J. Chemical in soybeans causes sexual dysfunctions in male rats. eHealthy News You Can Use, Mar. 26, 2003:www.mercola.com.

49. Whitaker, J. *Natural healing: what you're not being told.* Potomac, MD: Phillips Health, 2002.

50. "Soy: cutting through the confusion." *Consumer Reports,* July 2004:28–31.

51. Foreman, J. "Taking a closer look at soy." *Los Angeles Times,* June 14, 2004:F1.

52. Pratt, S, Matthews, C. *Superfoods*. New York: HarperCollins Publishers Inc., 2004.

53. Gaddi, A, Descovich, GC, Noseda, G, "Controlled evaluation of pantethine, a natural hypolipidemic compound, in patients with different forms of hyperlipoproteinemia." *Atherosclerosis* 1984;50(1): 73–83.

54. Arsenio L, Bodria, P, Magnati, G, et al. "Effectiveness of long-term treatment with pantethine in patients with dyslipidemia." *Clinical Therapeutics* 1986;8(5):537–45.

55. Binaghi, P, Cellina, G, Lo Cicero, G, et al. "Evaluation of the cholesterol-lowering effectiveness of pantethine in women in peri-menopausal age." *Minerva Medicina* 1990;81(6):475–9. Abstract

56. Qureshi AA, Sami SA, Salser WA, Khan FA. "Dose-dependent suppression of serum cholesterol by tocotrienol-rich fraction (TRF25) of rice bran in hypercholesterolemic humans." *Atherosclerosis* 2002;161(1):199–207.

57. Qureshi, AA, Bradlow, BA, Brace, L, et al. "Response of hypercholesterolemic subjects to administration of tocotrienols." *Lipids* 1995;30(12):1171–7.

58. Mustad, VA, Smith, CA, Ruey, PP, et al. "Supplementation with 3 compositionally different tocotrienol supplements does not improve cardiovascular disease risk factors in men and women with hypercholesterolemia." *American Journal of Clinical Nutrition* 2002;76(6):1237–43.

59. O'Byrne, D, Grundy, S, Packer, L, et al. "Studies of LDL oxidation following alpha-, gamma-, or delta-tocotrienyl acetate supplementation of hypercholesterolemic humans." *Free Radical Biology and Medicine* 2000;29(9):834–45.

60. Mensink, RP, van Houwelingen, AC, Kromhout, D, Hornstra, G. "A vitamin E concentrate rich in tocotrienols had no effect on serum lipids, lipoproteins, or platelet function in men with mildly elevated serum lipid concentrations." *American Journal of Clinical Nutrition* 1999;69(2):213–9.

61. Gilroy, CM, Steiner, JF, Byers, TB, et al. "Echinacea and truth in labeling." *Archives of Internal Medicine* 2003;163:699–704.

62. Sinatra, S, Sinatra, J. *Lower your blood pressure in eight weeks.* New York: Ballantine Books, 2003.

Chapter 5

1. Siguel, EN. *Essential Fatty Acids in Health and Disease.* Brookline, MA: Nutrek Press, 1994.

2. O'Keefe, JH Jr, Harris, WS. "From Inuit to implementation: omega-3 fatty acids come of age." *Mayo Clinic Proceedings* 2000; 75(6):607–14.

3. "Dietary supplementation with n-3 polyunsaturated fatty acids and vitamin E after myocardial infarction: results of the GISSI-Prevenzione trial." *Lancet* 1999;354(9177):447–55.

4. de Lorgeril, M, et al. "Dietary prevention of sudden cardiac death." *European Heart Journal* 2002;23:277–285.

5. Albert, CM, et al. "Blood Levels of Long-Chain N-3 Fatty Acids and the Risk of Sudden Death." *New England Journal of Medicine* 2002;346(15):1113–18.

6. Hu, FB, et al. "Fish and Omega-3 Fatty Acid Intake and Risk of Coronary Heart Disease in Women." *JAMA* 2002;287(14):1815–21.

7. Marchioli, R, et al. "Early Protection against Sudden Death by N-3 Polyunsaturated Fatty Acids after Myocardial Infarction." *Circulation* 2002;105:1897–1903.

8. Renaud, SC, Lanzmann-Petithory, D. "Coronary Heart Disease: Dietary Links and Pathogenesis." *Public Health and Nutrition* 2001: 459–74.

9. Simopoulos, AP. "Essential Fatty Acids in Health and Chronic Disease." *American Journal of Clinical Nutrition* 1999;70(suppl):560S-569S.

10. Demaison, L, Moreau, D. *Cellular and Molecular Life Science* 2002;59:463–477.

11. Sinatra, S. Coenzyme Q_{10}, Sept. 26 2002:http://www.drsinatra.com/index.asp.

12. Brody, JE. "Tip the Scale in Favor of Fish: The Healthful Benefits Await." *The New York Times,* July 29, 2003:nytimes.com.

13. Weil, A. Cardiovascular disease, June 6, 2003:www.drweil.com.

14. Sinatra, S. Health Email Report, 8/21/03.

15. "Mercury in seafood linked to infertility." Reuters Health, Sept. 24, 2002:www.reuters.com.

16. Mercola, J. Mercury in fish. www.mercola.com/2002/jun/5/toxic_waste.htm:3/3/2003.

17. Whitaker, J. *Sidestep Your Side Effects.* Potomac, MD: Phillips Health, 2002.

18. Wright, K. "B-vitamin linked to healthy hearts." *San Diego Union-Tribune,* 1/19/02:E1.

19. McCully, KS. "Homocysteine, folate, vitamin B_6, and cardiovascular disease." *JAMA* 1998;280:417.

20. Bazzano, LA, He, J, Ogden, LG, et al. "Dietary intake of folate and risk of stroke in U.S. men and women: NHANES I epidemiologic follow-up study." *Stroke* 2002;33:1183–1189.

21. Hackam, DG, Peterson, JC, Spence, JD. "What level of plasma homocysteine should be treated? Effects of vitamin therapy on progression of carotid atherosclerosis in patients with homocysteine levels above and below 14 micromoles/L." *American Journal of Hypertension* 2000;13(1 Pt1):105–10.

22. Rydlewicz A, Simpson JA, Taylor RJ, et al. "The effect of folic acid supplementation on plasma homocysteine in an elderly population." *QJM* 2002;95(1):27–35.

23. Hirschenbein, N. Personal communication, June 10, 2003.

24. Kannel, WB. "Cardioprotection: What is it? Who needs it?" Protection across the Cardiovascular Continuum, University of Cincinnati 2002:4–11.

25. Facts about Dietary Supplements. Office of Dietary Supplements, National Institutes of Health, Mar. 2001.

26. Topalov, V, Kovacevic, D, Topalov, A, et al. "Magnesium in cardiology." *Medicinski Pregled* [*Medical Review* (*Croatia*)] 2000;53:319–324, Abstract.

27. Carper, J. "Mighty magnesium: This overlooked nutrient fights against heart disease, pain and diabetes." USA Weekend, Aug. 30, 2002:http://usaweekend.com.

28. Oladapo, OO, F, AO. *African Journal of Medicine and Medical Science* 2000;29:265–268.

29. Wright, JV. *Nutrition & Healing*, March 2003:4.

30. Sinatra, S. *2003 Consumer's Guide to Rx and OTC Drugs.* Potomac MD: Phillips Health, 2003.

31. Rakel, R.E. *Conn's Current Therapy.* Philadelphia: W.B. Saunders Company, 1993.

Chapter 6

1. *Physicians' Desk Reference,* 57th Edition. Montvale, N.J.: Medical Economics Company, 2003.

2. American Society of Hospital Pharmacists. *American Hospital Formulary Service, Drug Information 2002.* Gerald K. McEvoy, Editor. Bethesda: 2002.

3. Jenkins, DJ, Kendall, CW, Marchie, A, et al. "Effects of a dietary portfolio of cholesterol-lowering foods vs. lovastatin on serum lipids and C-reactive protein." *JAMA* 2003;290:502–509.

4. Sylvester, B. "Ape diet" equals cholesterol drugs. UPI Science News, 7/25/2003.

5. Anderson, JW. "Diet first, then medication for hypercholesterolemia." *JAMA* 2003;290:531–533.

6. Haney, DQ (Associated Press). "Study finds Atkins diet may have surprising benefit on cholesterol." *San Diego Union-Tribune*, November 18, 2002.

7. Roberts WC. "Preventing and arresting coronary atherosclerosis." *American Heart Journal* 1995;130(3 Pt 1):580–600.

8. Noonan, D. "You want statins with that?" *Newsweek* 7/14/O3: 48–53.

9. Johnston, CS, Tjonn, SL, Swan, PD. "High-Protein, Low-Fat Diets Are Effective for Weight Loss and Favorably Alter Biomarkers in Healthy Adults1." *Journal of Nutrition* 2004;134:586–591.

10. Patrick, L, Uzick, M. "Cardiovascular disease: C-reactive protein and the inflammatory disease paradigm." *Alternative Medicine Review* 2001;6:248–271.

11. Trichopoulou, A, Costacou, T, Bamia, C, Trichopoulos, D. "Adherence to a Mediterranean Diet and Survival in a Greek Population." *New England Journal of Medicine* 2003;348:2599–2608.

12. Willett, WC. "Mediterranean Diet and Health." Pages 24–26 in: The Best of Experts Speak. Sacramento, ITServices: 2000.

13. Esselstyn, CB. "Becoming Heart Attack Proof." Cleveland Clinic Foundation:www.heartattackproof.com.

14. Ornish, D, Scherwitz, LW, Billings, JH, et al. "Intensive lifestyle changes for reversal of coronary heart disease." *JAMA* 1998;280(23):2001–7.

15. Ornish D. "Avoiding revascularization with lifestyle changes: The Multicenter Lifestyle Demonstration Project." *American Journal of Cardiology* 1998;82(10B):72T-76T.

16. Lakka, H, Laakosonen, DE, Lakka, TA, et al. "The metabolic syndrome and total and cardiovascular disease mortality in middle-aged men." *JAMA* 2002;288:2709–2716.

17. Wright, J. "Should you go low-carb?" *Nutrition & Healing*, June 2004;11:1–5.

18. Park, YW, et al. "The Metabolic Syndrome: Prevalence and Associated Risk Factor Findings in the US Population From the Third National Health and Nutrition Examination Survey, 1988–1994." *Archives of Internal Medicine* 2003;163:427–436.

19. Ford, ES, Giles, WH, Dietz, WH. "Prevalence of the metabolic syndrome in U.S. adults: findings from NHANES III." *JAMA* 2002;287:356–359.

20. Hoffman, R. Personal communication, July 18, 2004.

21. Baker, J. Personal communication, July 1, 2002.

22. Bravata, DM, Sanders, LS, Huang, J, et al. "Efficacy and safety of low-carbohydrate diet." *JAMA* 2003;289:1837–1850.

23. Foster, GD, et al. "A Randomized Trial of a Low-Carbohydrate

Diet for Obesity." *New England Journal of Medicine* 2003;348: 2082–2092.

24. "The Diet That Works." *The Wall Street Journal*, April 22, 2003: www.wsj.com.

25. Brody, JE. "Fear not that carrot, potato, or ear of corn." *The New York Times*, June 11, 2002.

26. Mirkin, G. Glycemic Load, 11/15/01:www.drmirkin.com/nutrition/9566.html.

27. Liu S. "Intake of refined carbohydrates and whole grain foods in relation to risk of type 2 diabetes mellitus and coronary heart disease." *Journal of the American College of Nutrition* 2002;21(4):298–306.

28. Willett W, Manson J, Liu S. "Glycemic index, glycemic load, and risk of type 2 diabetes." *American Journal of Clinical Nutrition* 2002;76(1):274S-80S.

29. Hallfrisch J, Facn, Behall, KM. "Mechanisms of the effects of grains on insulin and glucose responses." *American Journal of Clinical Nutrition* 2000;19(3 Suppl):320S-325S.

30. Liu, S. "Whole-grain foods, dietary fiber, and type 2 diabetes: searching for a kernel of truth." *American Journal of Clinical Nutrition* 2003;77:527–529.

31. Liu, S, Manson, JE, Stampfer, MJ, et al. "A prospective study of whole-grain intake and risk of type 2 diabetes mellitus n US women." *American Journal of Public Health* 2000;90(9):1409–1415.

32. Slavin, JL. "Mechanisms for the impact of whole grain foods on cancer risk." Journal of the *American College of Nutrition* 2000;19(3 Suppl):300S-307S.

33. La Vecchia, C, Chatenoud, L, Altieri, A, Tavani, A. "Nutrition and health: epidemiology of diet, cancer and cardiovascular disease in Italy." *Nutrition and Metabolism in Cardiovascular Disease* 2001;11(4 Suppl):10–15.

34. Liu, S, Sesso, HD, Manson, JE, et al. "Is intake of breakfast cereals related to total and cause-specific mortality in men?" *American Journal of Clinical Nutrition* 2003;77:594–599.

35. Periera, MA, Jacobs, DR, Pins, JJ, et al. "Effect of whole grains on insulin sensitivity in overweight hyperinsulinemic adults." *American Journal of Clinical Nutrition* 2000;75:848–55.

36. Brody, JE. "For unrefined healthfulness: whole grains." *The New York Times*, Mar. 4, 2003:www.nytimes.com.

37. Tufts University Health & Nutrition Letter, June 2003:21:8.

38. Hu, FB, Willett, WC. "Optimal diets for prevention of coronary heart disease." *JAMA* 2002;288:2569–2578.

39. Wolcott, WL. *The Metabolic Typing Diet*. New York: Doubleday, 2000.

40. Wolcott, WL. "Metabolic typing." eHealthy News You Can Use e-newsletter, Dec. 18, 2002;386:www.mercola.com.

41. Hellmich, N, Rubin, R. "Health guidelines: It's tough keeping up." *USA Today*, June 16, 2003:1A.

Chapter 7

1. Davis, W. "Cholesterol & Statin Drugs: separating hype from reality." *Life Extension Magazine*, Collector's Edition, Mar. 2005:114–124.

2. American Medical Association Council on Ethical and Judicial Affairs. *Code of Medical Ethics, 1998–1999 Edition*. American Medical Association, Chicago, IL.

3. Braddock, CH, Edwards, KA, Hasenberg, NM, Laidley, TL, Levinson, W. "Informed Decision Making in Outpatient Practice: Time to Get Back to Basics." *JAMA* 1999;282:2313–20.

ABOUT THE AUTHOR

Dr. Jay Cohen is a widely recognized expert on prescription medications and non-drug alternatives that work. Dr. Cohen is a Voluntary (Adjunct) Associate Professor of Family and Preventive Medicine and of Psychiatry at the University of California, San Diego. Dr. Cohen is also the Chairman of the Medical Advisory Committee of The Erythromelalgia Association.

Dr. Cohen graduated cum laude and the equivalent of Phi Beta Kappa from Ursinus College in 1967. He earned his medical degree at Temple University in 1971. After completing his internship, Dr. Cohen practiced general medicine, then conducted pain research at UCLA. He then completed a psychiatry residency at the University of California, San Diego, and practiced psychiatry and psychopharmacology until 1990.

Since 1990, Dr. Cohen has been conducting independent research in the area of general pharmacology. Specifically, Dr. Cohen has focused on the causes of medication side effects and sought solutions to solve this decades-long problem that is responsible for more than 100 deaths annually. Since 1996, Dr. Cohen has been publishing his findings in leading medical journals and major magazines. Dr. Cohen has published eight books. This is his fourth book on natural therapies for medical disorders.

Dr. Cohen has been featured on more than 100 radio programs across America including the "People's Pharmacy" and National Public Radio "Morning Edition." Dr. Cohen has spoken at conferences of patients, doctors, drug industry executives, malpractice attorneys, and at the U.S. Food and Drug Administration.

Dr. Cohen conducts his research independently. He has never accepted funding from the drug industry. Dr. Cohen performs his research and writing in Del Mar, CA.

INDEX

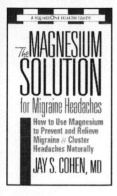

THE MAGNESIUM SOLUTION FOR MIGRAINE HEADACHES

How to Use Magnesium to Prevent and Relieve Migraine & Cluster Headaches Naturally

Jay S. Cohen, MD

More than 30 million people in North America suffer from migraine headaches. While a number of drugs are used to treat migraines, they come with a risk of side effects. But there is a safe alternative—magnesium. This guide shows how magnesium can treat migraines, and pinpoints the best types of magnesium to use and the proper dosage.

$5.95 • 96 pages • 4 x 7-inch mass paperback • ISBN 978-0-7570-0256-4

THE MAGNESIUM SOLUTION FOR HIGH BLOOD PRESSURE

How to Use Magnesium to Prevent & Relieve Hypertension Naturally

Jay S. Cohen, MD

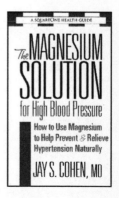

About 50 percent of Americans have hypertension. While many medications are available to combat this condition, they come with potential side effects. Fortunately, there is a remedy that is both safe and effective—magnesium. *The Magnesium Solution for High Blood Pressure* describes the best types of magnesium, explores appropriate dosage, and details the use of magnesium with hypertension meds.

$5.95 • 96 pages • 4 x 7-inch mass paperback • ISBN 978-0-7570-0255-7

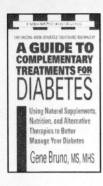

A GUIDE TO COMPLEMENTARY TREATMENTS FOR DIABETES

Using Natural Supplements, Nutrition, and Alternative Therapies to Better Manage Your Diabetes

Gene Bruno, MS, MHS

If you are among the 17 million American who have diabetes, you are probably working with a doctor to maintain an appropriate treatment program. But what if you could do more to improve your health? In *A Guide to Complementary Treatments for Diabetes,* Gene Bruno reveals natural ways to complement your current diabetes management. Unique in its approach, this book will help you assume an active role in your diabetes program and enjoy the greatest health possible.

$7.95 • 176 pages • 4 x 7-inch mass paperback • ISBN 978-0-7570-0322-6

NATURAL ALTERNATIVES TO NEXIUM, MAALOX, TAGAMET, PRILOSEC & OTHER ACID BLOCKERS

What to Use to Relieve Acid Reflux, Heartburn, and Gastric Ailments

Martie Whittekin, CCN

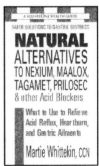

Written by Martie Whittekin, an experienced clinical nutritionist, this book examines the underlying causes of acid reflux. It also discusses how acid blockers work and how they can be damaging to long-term health. If you suffer from the pain of recurrent gastric upset, or if you are currently using an acid blocker, *Natural Alternatives to Nexium, Maalox, Tagamet, Prilosec & Other Acid Blockers* can make a profound difference in the quality of your life.

$7.95 • 160 pages • 4 x 7-inch mass paperback • ISBN 978-0-7570-0210-6

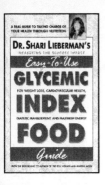

TRANSITIONS LIFESTYLE SYSTEM GLYCEMIC INDEX FOOD GUIDE
For Weight Loss, Cardiovascular Health, Diabetic Management, and Maximum Energy

Dr. Shari Lieberman

This book was designed as an easy-to-use guide to the glycemic index. The book first answers commonly asked questions, ensuring that you truly understand the GI and know how to use it. It then provides both the glycemic index and the glycemic load of hundreds of foods and beverages, including raw foods, cooked foods, and many combination and prepared foods. Whether you are interested in controlling your glucose levels to manage your diabetes, lose weight, increase your heart health, or simply enhance your well-being, *Transitions Lifestyle System Glycemic Index Food Guide* is the best place to start.

$7.95 • 160 pages • 4 x 7-inch mass paperback • ISBN 978-0-7570-0245-8

THE ACID-ALKALINE FOOD GUIDE
A Quick Reference to Foods & Their Effect on pH Levels

Dr. Susan E. Brown and Larry Trivieri, Jr.

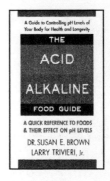

The Acid-Alkaline Food Guide is a complete resource for people who want to widen their food choices. The book begins by explaining how the acid-alkaline environment of the body is influenced by foods. It then presents a list of thousands of foods—single foods, combination foods, and even fast foods—and their acid-alkaline effects. *The Acid-Alkaline Food Guide* will quickly become the resource you turn to at home, in restaurants, and whenever you want to select a food that can help you reach your health and dietary goals.

$7.95 • 208 pages • 4 x 7-inch mass paperback • ISBN 978-0-7570-0280-9

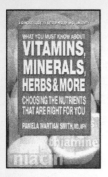

WHAT YOU MUST KNOW ABOUT VITAMINS, MINERALS, HERBS & MORE

Choosing the Nutrients That Are Right for You

Pamela Wartian Smith, MD, MPH

Almost 75 percent of your health and life expectancy is based on lifestyle, environment, and nutrition. Yet even if you follow a healthful diet, you are probably not getting all the nutrients you need to prevent disease. In *What You Must Know About Vitamins, Minerals, Herbs & More,* Dr. Pamela Smith explains how you can restore and maintain health through the wise use of nutrients.

$15.95 • 448 pages • 6 x 9-inch quality paperback • ISBN 978-0-7570-0233-5

JUICE ALIVE

The Ultimate Guide to Juicing Remedies

Steven Bailey, ND and Larry Trivieri, Jr.

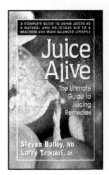

Juice Alive begins with a look at the history of juicing. It then examines the many components that make fresh juice truly good for you—good for weight loss and so much more. Next, it offers practical advice about the types of juices available, as well as buying and storing tips for produce. The second half of the book begins with an important chart that matches up common ailments with the most appropriate juices, followed by over 100 delicious juice recipes. Let *Juice Alive* introduce you to a world bursting with the incomparable tastes and benefits of fresh juice.

$14.95 • 272 pages • 6 x 9-inch quality paperback • ISBN 978-0-7570-0266-3